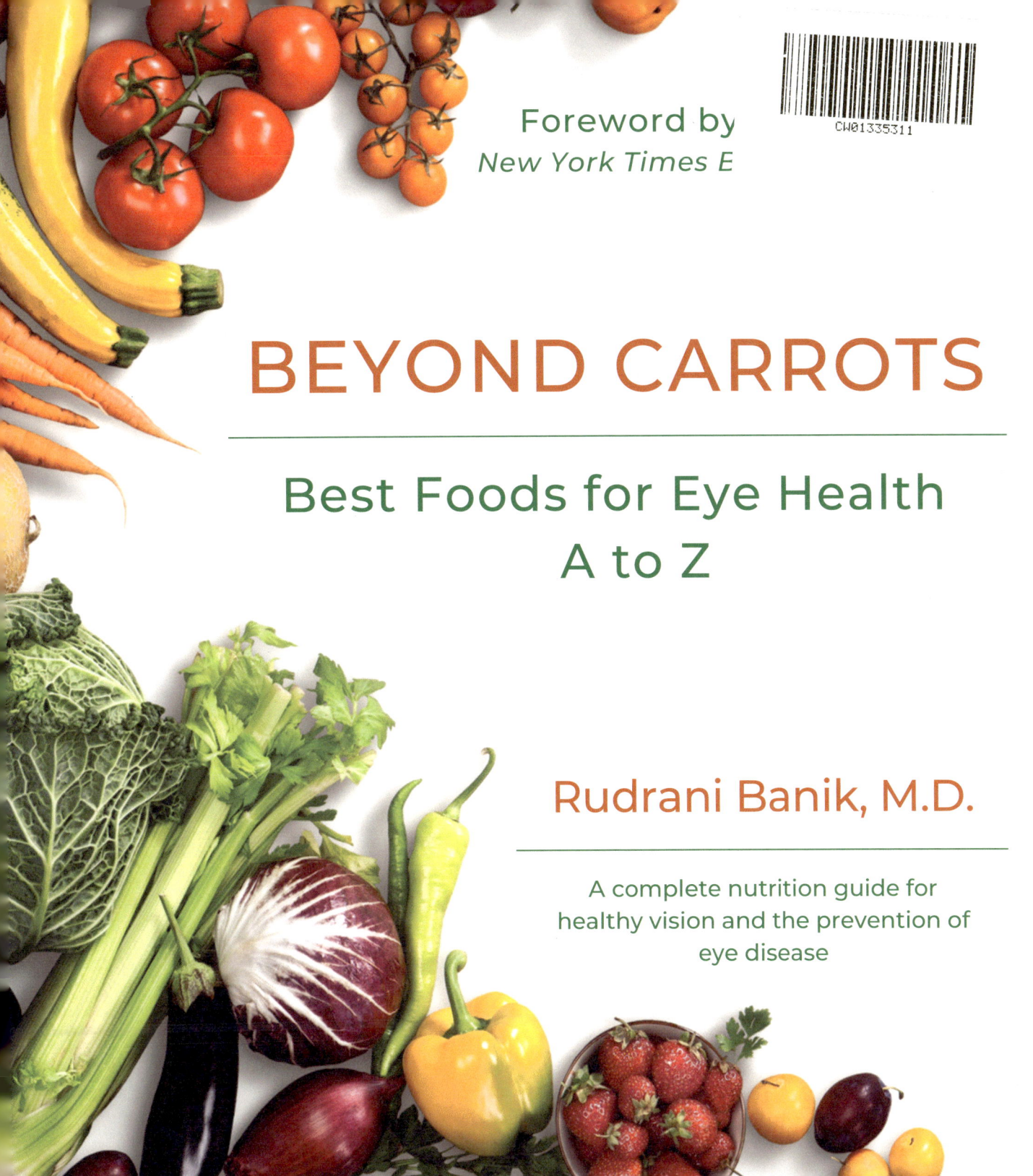

Foreword by
New York Times E

BEYOND CARROTS

Best Foods for Eye Health A to Z

Rudrani Banik, M.D.

A complete nutrition guide for healthy vision and the prevention of eye disease

Praise for 'Beyond Carrots'

"Dr. Rani Banik is a pioneer in Integrative Ophthalmology, a field in which nutritional and lifestyle choices are put at the forefront to maintain eye health. Her first book is a landmark contribution."
- Dr. Kellyann Petrucci, New York Times Best-Selling Author of *The Bone Broth Diet*

"Paradigm-shifting. By connecting the importance of nutrition with our eyes, Dr. Banik gives us key strategies to protect against vision loss. I love this book!"
- JJ Virgin, CNS CHFS, New York Times Best-Selling Author

"A must-read for anyone who cares about protecting their eyesight naturally using food as medicine."
- Jason Wachob, Founder & Co-CEO, mindbodygreen

"In 'Beyond Carrots,' Dr. Banik synthesizes her vast medical knowledge, clinical acumen, and personal life experience to create an encyclopedic compendium of nutritional pearls that empowers each of us to take control of our own visual health..."
- Paul A. Sidoti, M.D., Professor and Chair, New York Eye and Ear Infirmary of Mount Sinai

"Dr. Banik is a reliable purveyor of information about eye health. With her impeccable conventional credentials, as well as dedication to studying natural alternatives, she can truly lay claim to being America's foremost integrative ophthalmologist."
- Ronald Hoffman, M.D., Podcast Host, "Intelligent Medicine"

In 'Beyond Carrots,' Dr. Banik shares the groundbreaking science of keeping our eyes healthy with food. For anyone that cares about their vision, Dr. Banik's practical and delicious recommendations are crucial and will go a long way towards keeping your eyes healthy and strong as they age."
- Max Lugavere, NYT Best-Selling Author of *Genius Foods*; Health and Science Journalist

"...Dr. Rani Banik's first book is a landmark contribution. I'm excited for her message about protecting eyesight naturally using food as medicine can be delivered to as many people as possible."
- Dr. Rupy Aujla, MBBS, BSc, MRCGP, Founder and Podcast Host, "The Doctor's Kitchen"

"Finally! 'Beyond Carrots' is the comprehensive, deliciously easy resource our patients need to nourish their eyes and protect their vision. Dr. Banik is my go-to resource for practitioner and patient education..."
- Ashley Koff RD, Founder, The Better Nutrition Program

"This first book by Dr. Rudrani Banik, 'Beyond Carrots,' is a thorough science-based masterpiece revealing the role of the most important nutrients essential for keeping your eyes in good health. It will change the lives of many people who will read the book!"
- Gennady Landa, M.D., Assistant Professor, New York Eye and Ear Infirmary of Mount Sinai

"Dr. Rani Banik is a brilliant thought leader... In 'Beyond Carrots' she synthesizes the latest data from the literature and her own experience as a researcher and clinician. Her recommendations will surely improve all of our eye health through easy-to-follow and delicious recommendations. A must-read for everyone!"
    - Gary Goldman, MD, IFMCP, Faculty, Weill Medical College of Cornell University;
      Faculty, Institute for Functional Medicine

"Dr. Rani Banik is a rare find... She is forging the way in Integrative Ophthalmology, a field in which nutritional and lifestyle choices are put at the forefront to maintain eye health."
    - Dana G. Cohen, MD, Co-Author of *Quench*

"Eyes are not just the window to the soul, but also to our brain... I interviewed Dr. Rudrani Banik on Dr. Berkson's Best Health Radio... Dr. Banik shared pearl after pearl on how to keep seeing and thinking clearly... Most ophthalmologists don't know this stuff, but now you will!"
    - Dr. Devaki Lindsey Berkson, Author of *SEXY BRAIN* and *Safe Hormones, Smart Women*

"Brilliant! This is a must-read book to "look" and feel good! ... digital eyestrain is becoming alarmingly prevalent, and Dr. Banik beautifully shows readers how to take care of their eyes with a healthy diet."
    - Dr. Krista Burns DC, DHA, Founder of the American Posture Institute

"...Whether you have an existing eye condition or are looking to prevent one from developing, Dr. Banik's book 'Beyond Carrots' is a must-read. It's great to see a book that discusses all the different nutrients needed to have optimal eye health and the specific foods you need to eat to get them."
    - Eric Osansky, DC, IFMCP, Podcast Host, "Save My Thyroid Podcast"

"Everything in the body is connected, and what we eat is one of the most important factors for our health. Our eyes are no different. In this beautifully written and illustrated book, Dr. Banik explains exactly how to get and keep our eyes healthy through one of the most powerful tools - nutrition..."
    - Inna Topiler CNS, MS, Founder of Complete Nutrition And Wellness; Podcast Host, "Health
      Mysteries Solved"

"What an empowering guide for eye health! It's short yet packed with helpful information. Dr. Banik makes eye nutrition easy to understand and implement."
    - Eileen Laird, Author of *Healing Mindset*

"A must-read for anyone who cares about protecting their eyesight naturally using food as medicine."
    - Regan Jones, RDN, Creator and Podcast Host, "This Unmillennial Life Podcast"

"Since interviewing Dr. Rudrani for my Brave New Girl podcast, I have been so excited to read her new book 'Beyond Carrots'... The book is written clearly and is easy to follow, with colourful photos that make her nourishing nutritional advice inviting and inspiring. This is an eye-bible for life."
    - Lou Hamilton, Founder & Creative Director at Silk Studios; Podcast Host, "Brave New Girl"

Notices & Disclaimers

Disclaimers / Legal Information

All rights reserved. No part of this book may be reproduced, stored in a retrieval system or transmitted in any form or by any means, without the prior written permission of the author/publisher, except in the case of brief quotations for the purpose of writing critical articles or reviews.

Notice of Liability

The author and publisher have made every effort to ensure the accuracy of the information herein. However, the information contained in this book is presented without warranty, either express or implied.

Trademark Notice

Rather than indicating every occurrence of a trademarked name as such, this book uses the names only in an editorial fashion and to the benefit of the trademark owner with no intention of infringement of the trademark.

Copyright Information

©2023 Rudrani Banik, M.D.

Book design and layout by Lylah Patel.

Photographs by Canva under Content License Agreement.

https://rudranibanikmd.com/beyondcarrots

Contents

Dedication..i

Foreword by Frank Bruni...ii

Preface- A Message from Dr. Banik...iii

Part I - The Nutrients for Healthy Eyes..1

Part II- Therapeutic Foods for Eye Health A to Z.............................28

Part III - Eye-Healthy Recipes...69

Part IV - Supplements for Healthy Eyes..89

Additional Resources..113

Acknowledgments...118

References..119

About the Author...146

*This book is dedicated to my parents,
Dr. Rathindra Nath and Mrs. Kalyani Banik,
to whom I owe so very much,*

*and also to my uncle,
the late Mr. Swapan Kumar Banik,
who showed me the power
of nutrition and healthy living.*

Foreword

In terms of both our physical and our spiritual well-being, there's perhaps nothing as devastating as feeling powerless. There's also nothing as misguided. While we're all at the mercy of fate to some extent, those last three words are a crucial qualifier. We have tools and strategies with which we can potentially lower the odds of trouble ahead, minimize the toll of whatever befalls us, safeguard those aspects of our health on the periphery of the ailment in question and manage our emotional response. We're pilots as much as we are passengers, and the best doctors empower us with that understanding.

Rudrani Banik is one of those doctors. I know that not only from reading what she's written, following her social media posts and seeing her on television. I know that because during a profoundly challenging medical odyssey of my own, I found myself in her care. I'd had a kind of stroke in my right optic nerve, had lost much of the vision in that eye and was enrolled in two successive clinical trials of possible treatments, the first of which involved monthly injections in the affected eye and the second of which involved twice-weekly, self-administered injections in my belly or one of my thighs for six months. I'd never imagined being put through anything like that. I was often scared. I was less so thanks to Dr. Banik, who helped guide me through my trials in more ways than one.

She didn't and doesn't focus on what has irrevocably happened. She's concerned with thinking and planning ahead. She's interested in what each of us can control. This book is a testament to that.

While it's specifically about eye health and a regimen of prudent and pleasurable eating that may ward off disease, it's generally about taking charge and taking responsibility. It's about agency. It's about potency. Her principal vocabulary may be that of the refrigerator and the pantry – of cruciferous vegetables and aromatic herbs – but her message and meaning apply well beyond breakfast, lunch and dinner.

And the benefits of her counsel transcend the realm of vision. She vividly communicates something that most of us know but too frequently and easily ignore: Our bodies serve us only as well as we serve them, and what we get out of them reflects what we put into them. Every decision that we make should be a considered one, because every decision counts. That's an excellent philosophy for eating. It's an equally good one for life.

Frank Bruni
Professor, Duke University
Contributing Writer, New York Times
New York Times Best-Selling Author

Preface- A Message from Dr. Rudrani Banik

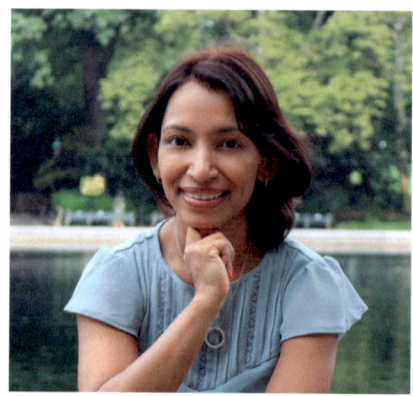

Food is medicine. What you put in your mouth has a tremendous impact on the health of your body, especially your visual system.

If your diet consists of simple sugars, unhealthy fats, and processed foods, your body will be predisposed to health conditions such as diabetes, cardiovascular disease, and inflammatory states that may damage your vision.

If your diet consists of foods rich in antioxidants, vitamins, minerals, healthy fats, and anti-inflammatory nutrients, your body (and your eyes!) will be equipped to fight and prevent disease.

I discovered this vital connection between food and optimal health the hard way. Unfortunately, I had little education on nutrition during medical school or my training as an ophthalmologist and neuro-ophthalmologist. It wasn't until I was debilitated by a health issue that I finally paid attention to nutrition and learned about the power of healthy food choices.

Doctor, Heal Thyself

I have a confession. Despite being a physician, I followed an incredibly unhealthy lifestyle for most of my adult life. As a medical student and young doctor, I worked long hours in a high-stress environment, survived on pizza, ice cream, and 8-12 caffeinated diet beverages a day, and slept 4-5 hours per night. I ate mainly processed foods, with hardly any fresh vegetables or fruits. I believed I would be immune to any consequences of these unhealthy habits. Eventually, they caught up with me.

In my early 40s, I developed excruciating migraines. I was plagued by daily headaches, light and sound sensitivity, brain fog, digestive issues, vertigo, and visual snow syndrome. For years, I lived in a zombie-like daze.

Looking back, I don't know how I managed - waking up with stabbing pain, getting my daughter ready for school, going to work, taking care of complex neuro-ophthalmic patients, teaching, operating, conducting research, and running a household - all with a non-stop migraine. Worse, none of the drugs prescribed by my doctors came close to easing my pain. After years of suffering, I desperately needed a different solution.

I then stumbled upon functional medicine, an integrative approach to health that aims to restore function and balance within the body's systems. Under the paradigm of functional medicine, the root cause of a chronic health issue is identified, such as:

- nutrient deficiency
- food intolerance
- inefficient energy production or metabolism
- high toxin load
- gut issue
- immune dysregulation
- latent infection or inflammation
- hormonal imbalance or
- any combination thereof

Once found, the root cause is addressed via personalized treatment strategies based on therapeutic diets, botanicals, supplements, and lifestyle modification. To learn more about functional medicine, please visit my website, *www.rudranibanikmd.com/beyondcarrots*.

My healing journey through functional medicine helped me address the root causes of my migraines - nutritional deficiencies, high toxin load, gut issues, and, most importantly, chronic stress. The therapeutic dietary and lifestyle changes I instituted to correct these issues impacted my life and career at a foundational level. Once empowered to manage my migraines via a functional medicine approach, I felt immensely better. I then applied similar treatment strategies for my patients, first for migraine and then for vision and neurologic issues.

The results I saw in my patients were astounding! Patients with poorly controlled diabetes stabilized their blood sugars. Patients with high blood pressure or cholesterol improved their numbers and decreased their dependence on medications. Patients with vision-threatening conditions also benefited. I witnessed patients with macular degeneration stop progressing, others with severe dry eye reverse their symptoms, and those with inflammatory eye conditions such as uveitis improve.

Healthy nutritional choices were the cornerstone of these positive vision and health outcomes. This epiphany I had stumbled upon through functional medicine turned around my health and the health of countless patients. I realized I needed to share this nutritional advice with the world and help people like you learn about the power of nutrition to protect and preserve their vision.

Who is this Book For?

I designed this book to make it easy for you to integrate what could be a complex subject - nutrition for preventing and treating visual conditions - into your daily life. You can benefit from this information if you:

- use screens all day and suffer from digital eye strain, dry eye, or light sensitivity.

- have been diagnosed with an early stage of cataract, glaucoma, or macular degeneration, or have a family history and want to prevent vision loss.

- are diabetic or pre-diabetic and want to prevent diabetic retinopathy.

- are the parent of a child who complains of blurred vision or headaches.

- are the child or caretaker of someone with glaucoma, cataract, or macular degeneration.

- want to be proactive to maintain your precious eyesight and continue reading, driving, using devices, and seeing your loved ones' faces into your golden years!

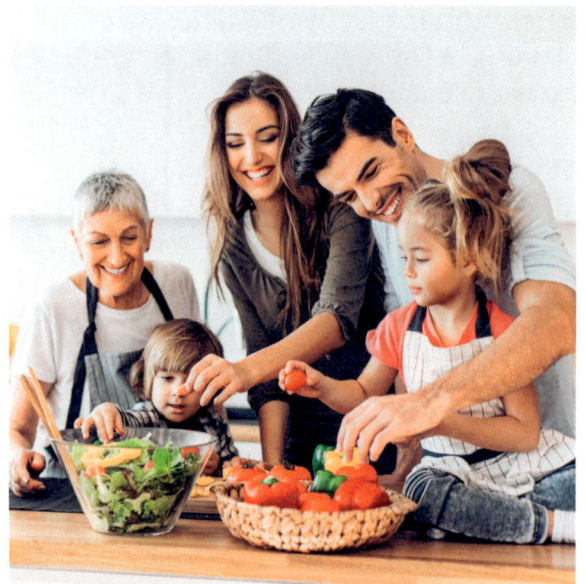

If you see yourself in any of the above scenarios, you will benefit from the nutrients, foods, and strategies in this book.

To get the most benefit, I invite you to take the Nutrition Eye-Q Test. After answering simple questions about your medical and eye history, current diet, and lifestyle habits, you will receive a personalized report. This report will outline which nutrients and foods highlighted in this book you should focus on to keep your eyes healthy.

To take the free online Nutrition Eye-Q Test, simply scan this QR code with your smartphone camera:

v

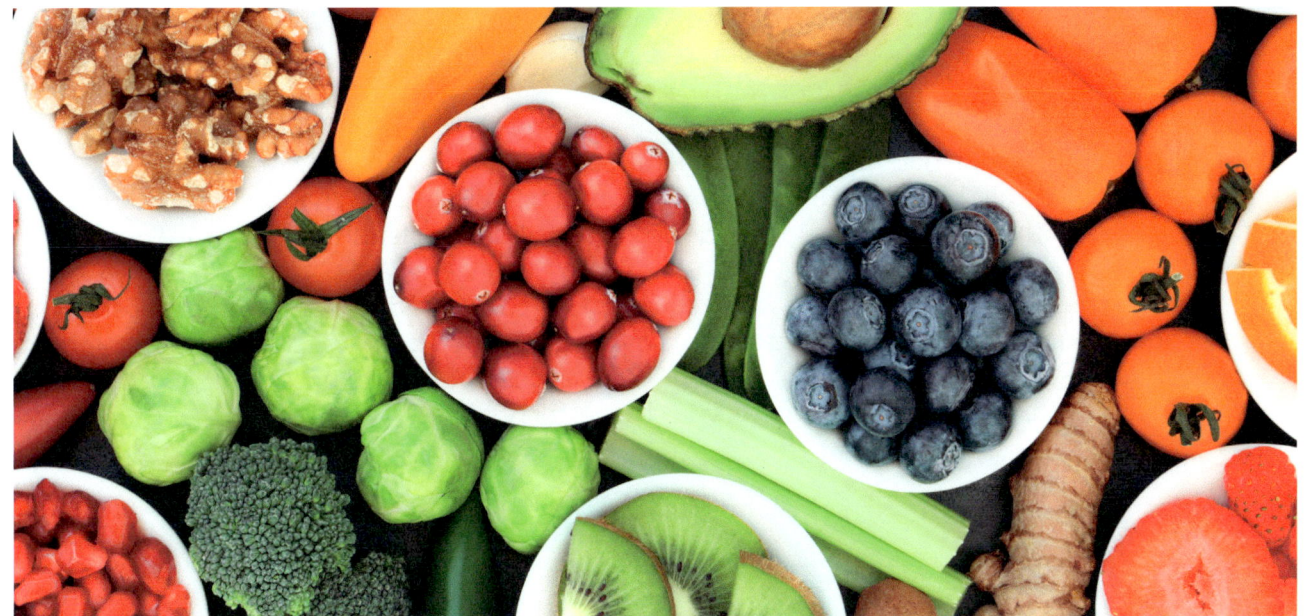

What's in this Book?

In **Part I, The Nutrients for Healthy Eyes**, you'll learn about the 30+ nutrients vital for vision, how to best incorporate them into your diet, and the specific nutrients needed by different parts of the eye that may help prevent disease.

In **Part II, Therapeutic Foods for Eye Health A to Z,** you'll be introduced to many foods rich in these eye health nutrients. These foods are carefully curated to provide the spectrum of nutrients your eyes need. Remember that this book is intended to serve as a general guide. Please adjust or swap foods if you have specific dietary needs or restrictions.

In **Part III, Eye-Healthy Recipes**, you will get a sneak peek into some of my favorite recipes that include multiple foods that support your eye health. This is a sample of the many delicious and nutritious recipes you can find in "The Beyond Carrots Cookbook," a recipe guide available for additional purchase that serves as a companion to this book.

Finally, in **Part IV, Supplements for Healthy Eyes**, you'll discover which supplements you should take for your eyes to fill in the nutritional gaps in your diet. You'll also learn about the published scientific research on supplements for eye health, and the shortcomings of some of these studies.

In case medical jargon may make you feel overwhelmed, don't worry. I wrote this book to be understandable to anyone. My goal is for you to pick up this book and, within an hour or two, have the tools you need to begin eating for healthy vision.

If you'd like a deeper explanation of some of the topics I discuss in this book or would like to explore more foods that benefit your eyes, I offer several free eBooks - "What are Integrative and Functional Medicine," "Eye Anatomy 101," and "Best Foods For Eye Health - A to Z Supplement."

You may find these useful resources that are companions to 'Beyond Carrots' via my website, *https://rudranibanikmd.com/beyondcarrots* or scan the QR code below and click on the tile that says "Download Free Resources." To unlock your FREE access, be sure to enter the secret word from the book, which is the food that starts with the letter 'V.'

You can access additional resources to help you implement the nutritional strategies described in this book. To maximally and optimally support your eye health through the power of nutrition, consider purchasing the Beyond Carrots Toolkit. This digital toolkit contains "The Beyond Carrots Meal Planner," "The Beyond Carrots Recipe Guide," and "The Beyond Carrots Grocery List." There are also vegetarian and vegan versions of the meal planner included in the toolkit.

To order the Toolkit, visit my website or scan the QR code above and click on the tile that says "Beyond Carrots Toolkit."

It is my hope that through the 'Beyond Carrots' series, you will be empowered with the nutritional strategies you need to keep your vision strong and healthy for a lifetime.

May these nutrients, foods, and recipes be a feast for your eyes!

To your eye health,

Dr. Rani Banik

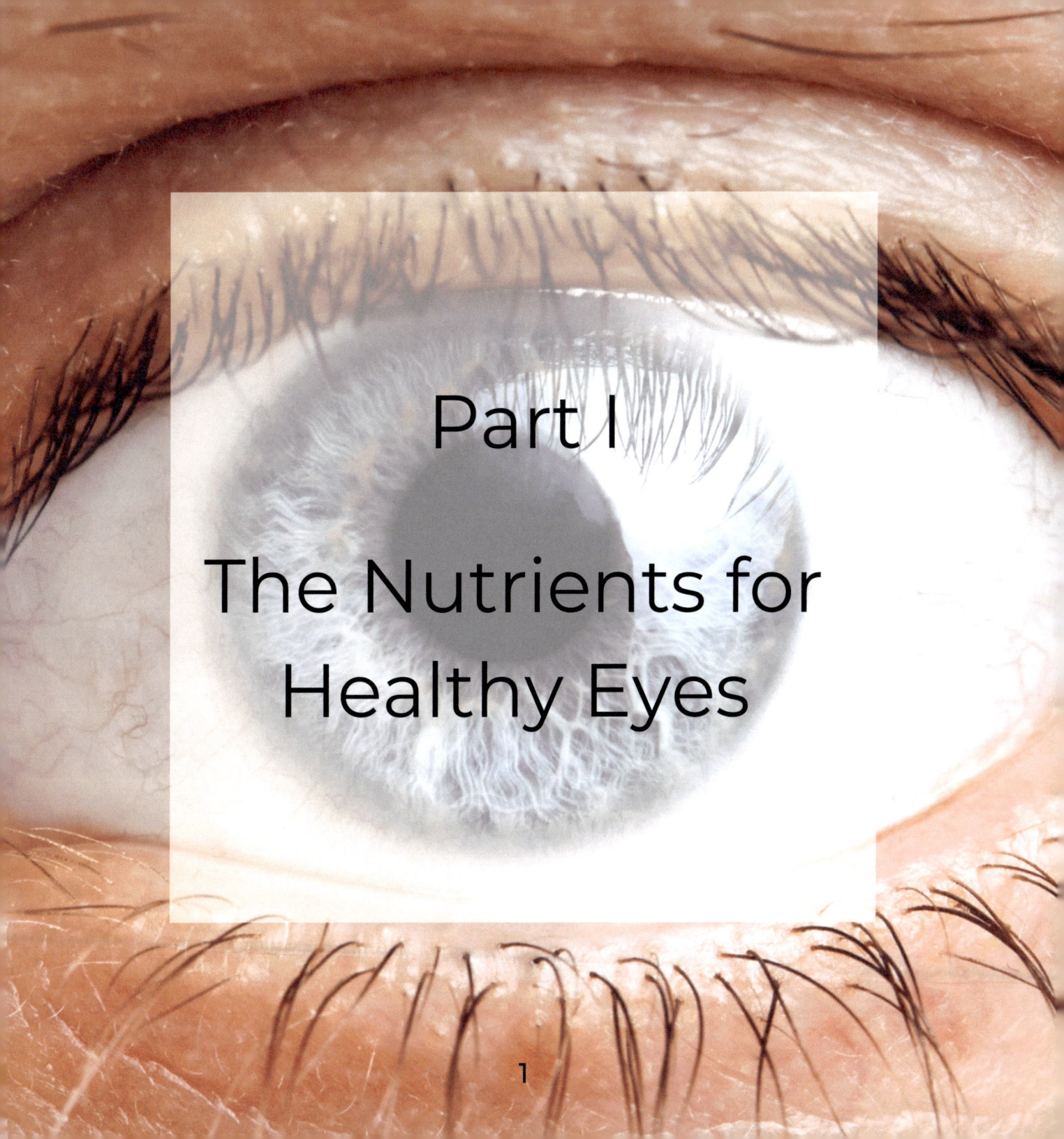

Part I

The Nutrients for Healthy Eyes

Of the five senses, most people would agree that vision is the most precious. Losing your vision or even the thought of losing your vision can be scary. This is true even if it's not your vision you're worried about but that of a loved one.

There is good news: you and your loved ones can protect your vision against common conditions such as dry eye, macular degeneration, cataracts, and glaucoma armed with eye-smart nutrition.

When it comes to nutrition for the eyes, one of the most common questions my patients ask is, "Dr. Banik, is it true that carrots are good for eyesight? Or is that a myth my parents told me to make me eat my veggies?"

Fortunately, the benefits of carrots for eye health are NOT a myth. Carrots are a rich source of a nutrient called beta-carotene. The body converts beta carotene into vitamin A. Vitamin A is essential to prevent night blindness and dry eye.

However, carrots are not the only food needed to keep your eyes seeing clearly, and vitamin A is not the only nutrient needed for healthy vision. The reality is that carrots and vitamin A are the tips of the iceberg for maintaining excellent eyesight.

For optimal vision health, you need to go beyond carrots!

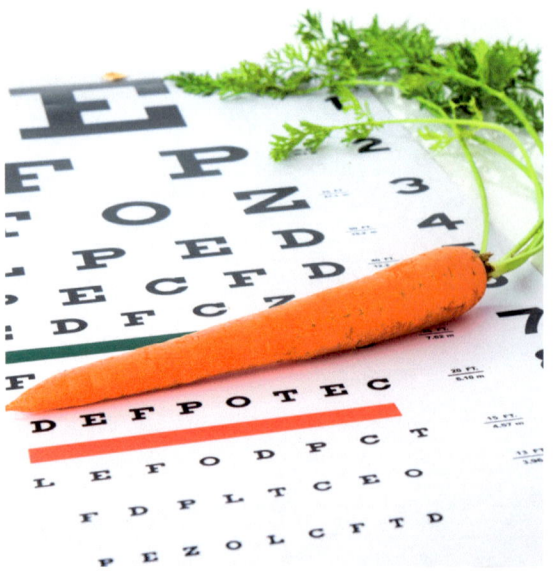

Your eyes need a wide variety of nutrients – vitamins, minerals, antioxidants, amino acids, fats, and polyphenols to maintain their healthy structure and optimal function.

If you total all the nutrients your eyes require, they can add up to 30 or more! Though this may feel overwhelming, again, there is good news -

Foods that you already know, and may even already be eating, are the single most powerful tool you can use to keep your vision strong. Fortunately, nature has already provided you with these foods. Now it's up to you to make the critical dietary choices to support your eyesight.

The 30+ Nutrients Your Eyes Need

What are these thirty nutrients your eyes need? Let's divide them into three categories:

- energy nutrients — fuel the powerful engine of your visual system
- antioxidants — help repair damaged cells
- anti-inflammatory nutrients — combat inflammation

Now let's take a dive deeper into each category.

Energy

Your eye, despite its small size, has high energy requirements. In other words, your eye is metabolically very active. Along with the brain, the eye has the highest metabolic rate in the entire body.

Why does an organ the size of a golf ball need so much energy to function?

The eye continually collects light rays and transforms this light energy into electrical energy. Moreover, the eye has over forty components that work in concert to process light energy, allowing for clear vision.

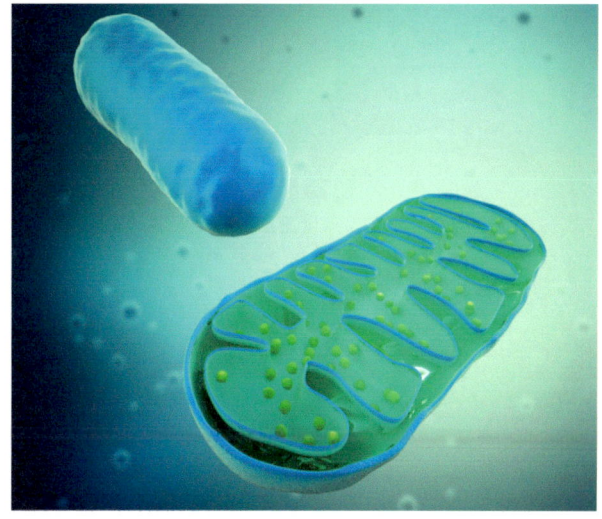

To support optimal energy production by your eye, you need to ensure a plentiful supply of nutrients to feed your mitochondria.

If you remember back to biology class, mitochondria are the energy powerhouses or factories within your cells.

They are tiny organelles responsible for breaking down the food molecules (such as carbohydrates, proteins, or fats) to produce energy. Your body could not function without your mitochondria.

The chemical processes by which mitochondria extract energy from food are quite complex and beyond the scope of this book. Suffice it to say that there is a range of nutrients, including vitamins, minerals, amino acids, and other molecules, that are necessary.

Below is a list of the many nutrients necessary for optimal mitochondrial function.

Vitamin B1 (Thiamine)	Carnitine (an amino acid)
Vitamin B2 (Riboflavin)	Taurine (an amino acid)
Vitamin B3 (Niacin)	L-arginine (an amino acid)
Vitamin B5 (Pantothenic Acid)	Iron (a mineral)
Vitamin B6 (Pyridoxine)	Zinc (a mineral)
Vitamin B7 (Biotin)	Magnesium (a mineral)
Vitamin B9 (Folate)	Manganese (a mineral)
Coenzyme Q10 (CoQ10)	Copper (a mineral)
Vitamin C (ascorbic acid)	Selenium (a mineral)
Vitamin E (tocopherol)	Alpha lipoic acid (ALA)

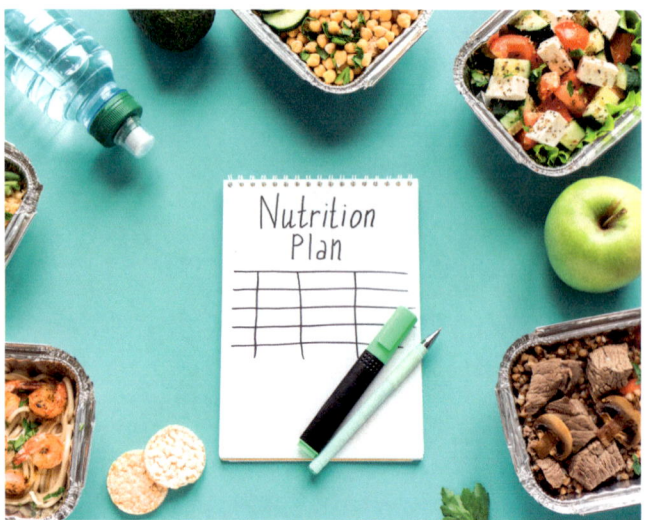

If you count them up, you will see that at least twenty nutrients are necessary for optimal mitochondrial energy production alone! If you feed your mitochondria with the foods richest in these nutrients, you will optimize energy production to support your eye's high metabolic needs.

It is important to note that some of these nutrients can be manufactured by our bodies, though most cannot. The nutrients that our bodies cannot make internally are considered "essential," meaning they must be obtained from our diet or supplements.

Antioxidants

Here's a fun fact- did you know that your eye has over forty components? Many of these structures are delicate and highly vulnerable to damage.

Damage to your eyes may occur from a variety of causes -

- waste products from energy metabolism
- high energy light rays such as ultraviolet (UV) or blue light wavelengths
- nutrient deficiencies
- toxins

Taken together, these types of damage are called "oxidative stress." You may be familiar with the term oxidation. The most well-recognized example of oxidation in nature is when the metal iron is exposed to oxygen and water. The result is the creation of rust.

But what happens when there is oxidation in the body, or better yet, in the eye? The result is a biological form of "rusting" that may ultimately lead to the dysfunction of cells and even cell death.

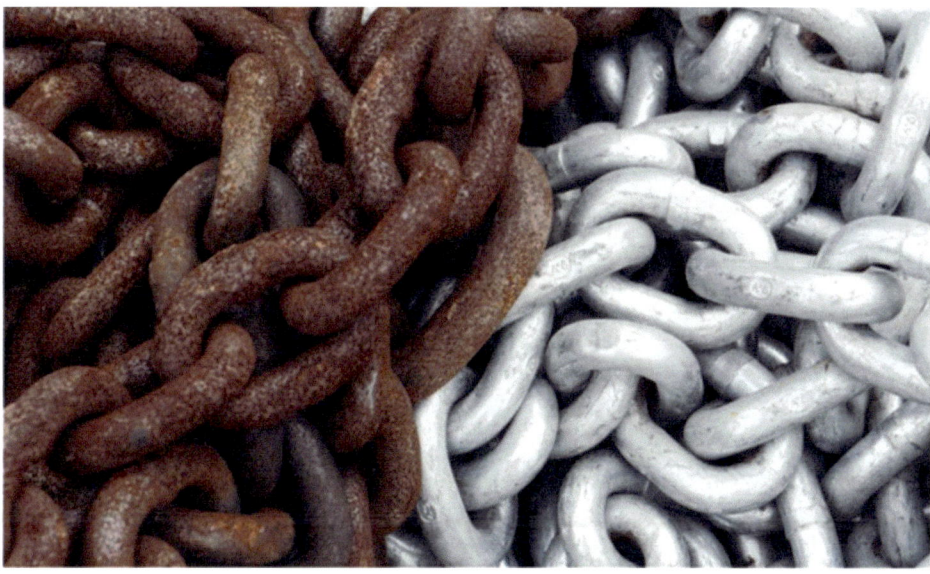

Before discussing oxidative damage further, let me first explain the concept of free radicals. If you remember back to chemistry class, free radicals are oxygen-containing molecules with an uneven number of electrons.

Electrons prefer to be paired, and because free radicals have unpaired electrons, the molecules are unstable. Free radicals, therefore, attempt to "steal" electrons from other molecules to stabilize themselves.

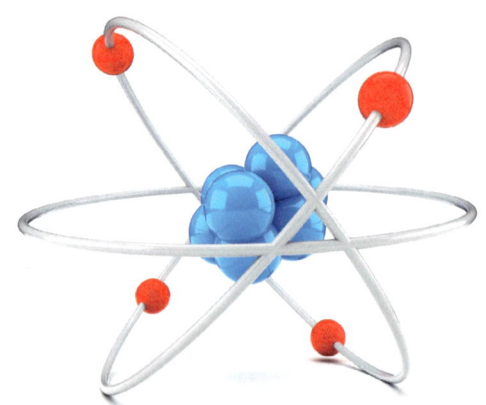

Free radicals can steal electrons from DNA (our genetic code), proteins, and fats, thus making these donor molecules unstable. This process is called oxidation.

If oxidation occurs on a large scale, a chain of chemical reactions can be triggered inside a cell, ultimately leading to loss of function and possibly even cell death.

Antioxidants are molecules that fight oxidative damage. Antioxidants tend to be large and can donate an electron to a free radical without making themselves unstable.

Antioxidants thus neutralize free radicals and stabilize them without causing damage to other molecules. Therefore, antioxidants are the defense mechanism of cells.

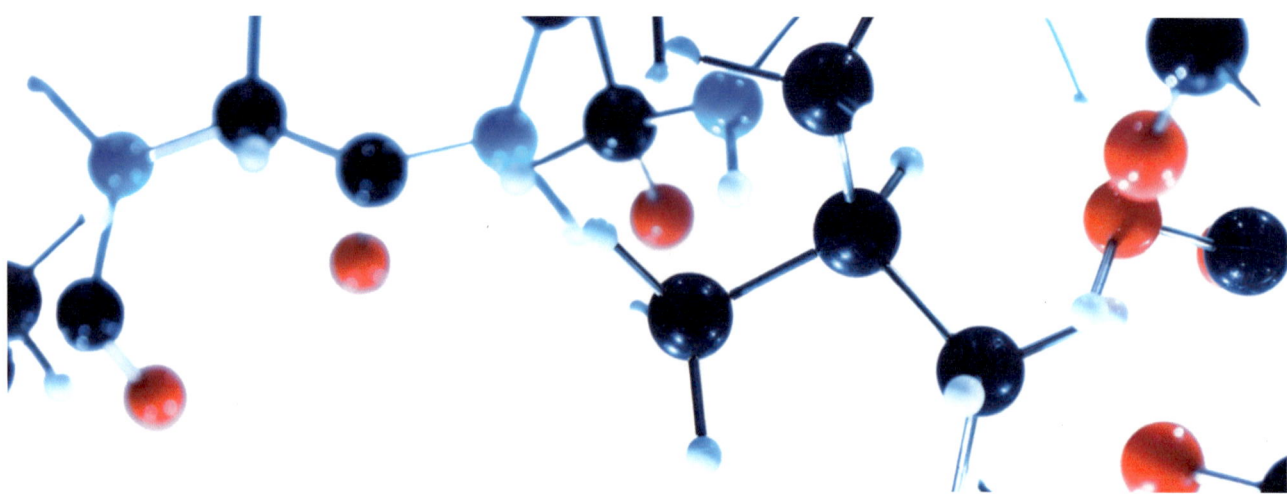

If the concept of free radicals and antioxidants seem foreign, consider this analogy-

imagine that a free radical is a car with a flat tire. Since it has only three wheels, the car is unstable.

This car desperately needs a fourth wheel, so it tries to steal a wheel from another vehicle.

But if it takes a wheel from another four-wheeled vehicle, the free radical car will make that vehicle unstable, likely causing an accident.

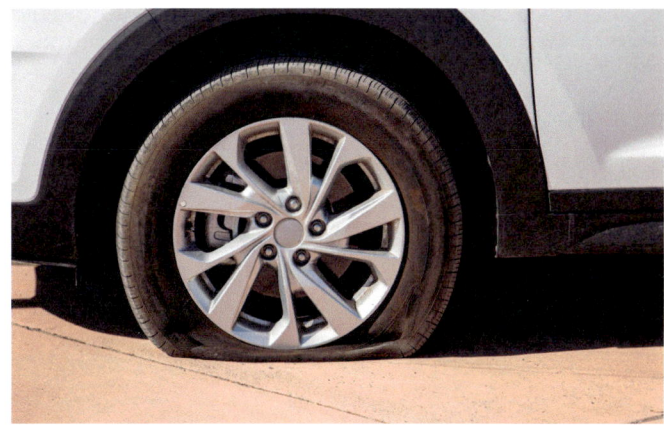

Along comes an 18-wheeler tractor-trailer. The 18-wheeler can donate one of its back wheels to the three-wheeled car without becoming too unstable

Thus, in this example, the 18-wheeler (the antioxidant) can stabilize the 3-wheeled car (the free radical) and protect other vehicles on the road from losing any of their wheels.

Of course, this is a simplistic view of oxidative damage that is not reality-based, but it helps get the point across.

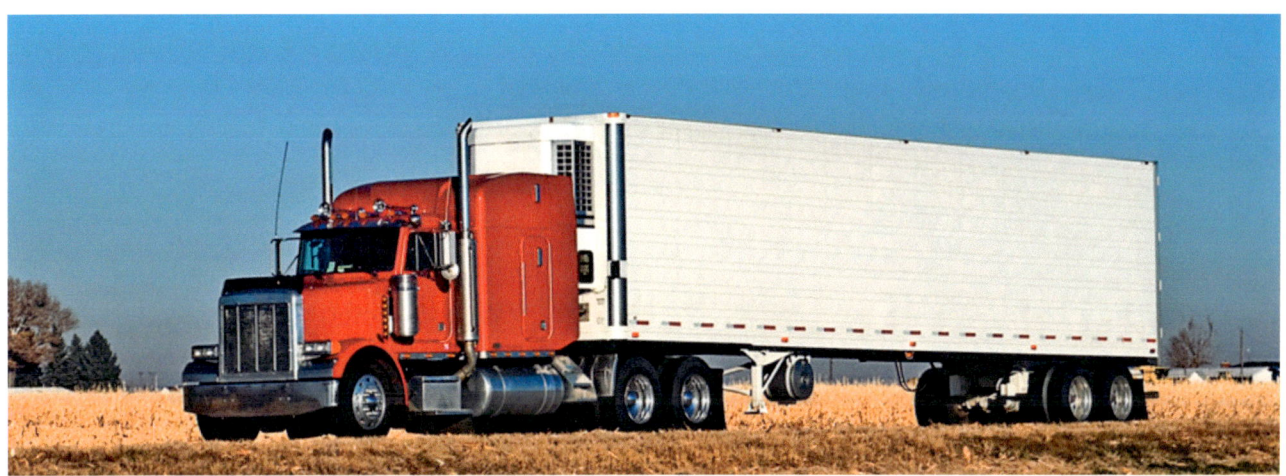

Not all oxidation in the body is harmful; oxidation is a necessary physiologic process. Free radicals can help your body fight off invaders such as bacteria and viruses that cause disease when your cells function correctly. However, oxidative damage occurs when there is an imbalance between too many free radicals and insufficient antioxidants.

Oxidative damage has been associated with many chronic health issues, some of which are more common with aging, such as:

- High Blood Pressure
- Diabetes
- Atherosclerosis (hardening of blood vessels)
- Heart Disease
- Inflammation
- Neurodegenerative Disease (Alzheimer's and Parkinson's)
- Cancer

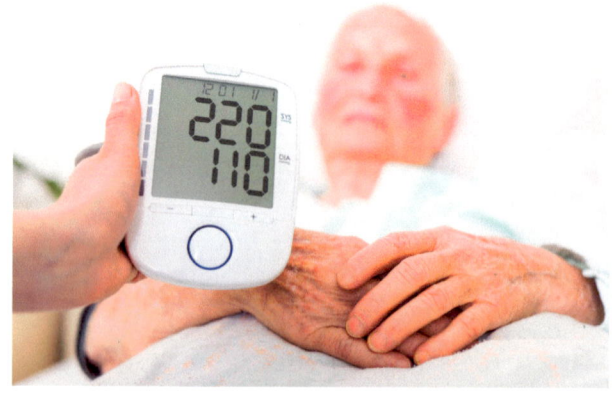

It is no surprise that the many delicate structures within the eye are susceptible to oxidative stress. Many eye diseases that commonly appear with aging, such as cataracts, glaucoma, and macular degeneration, all begin with oxidative damage.

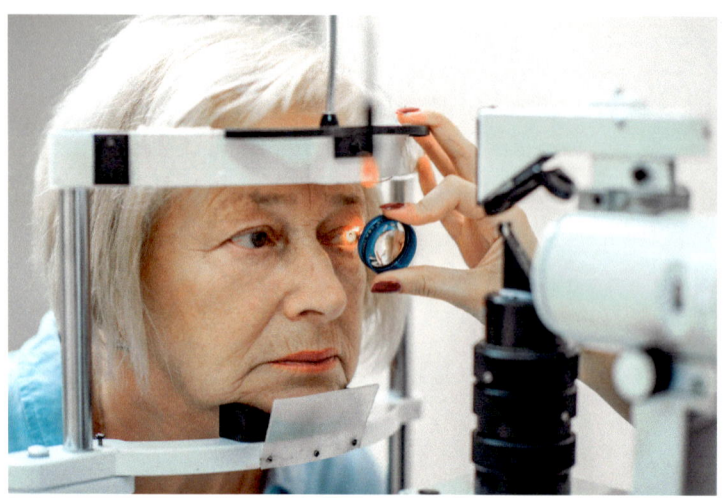

To add insult to injury, oxidative damage in your eye can prevent your mitochondria from functioning correctly, thus making energy production inefficient.

Inefficient mitochondria generate more free radicals as by-products, creating a vicious cycle of oxidative damage and mitochondrial dysfunction.

What are the best nutrients to fight oxidative stress in the eye?

Below is a list of the most potent antioxidant nutrients essential to protect your vision:

Vitamin A	Glutathione
Vitamin C (ascorbic acid)	N-acetyl cysteine (NAC)
Vitamin E (tocopherol)	Alpha lipoic acid (ALA)
Macular carotenoids - Lutein Zeaxanthin Meso-Zeaxanthin	Polyphenols - Bioflavonoids Resveratrol Tannins
Astaxanthin	

Note that some of these nutrients, such as vitamin C, vitamin E, and alpha-lipoic acid, are also found in the list for mitochondrial energy production noted in the previous section.

Luckily, there is some overlap in what your eyes need and the roles these nutrients play in supporting your vision!

To go further, there are antioxidant compounds known as bioflavonoids, a subset of the polyphenol category mentioned above. Bioflavonoids are abundant in nature as plant-derived compounds, with over 4,000 different types identified.

Bioflavonoids function as potent antioxidants, and several have been shown in research studies to protect your eye's delicate structures.

The bioflavonoids that are most important for your eye health include:

- Quercetin
- Anthocyanins
- Apigenin
- Epigallocatechin-3-gallate (EGCG)

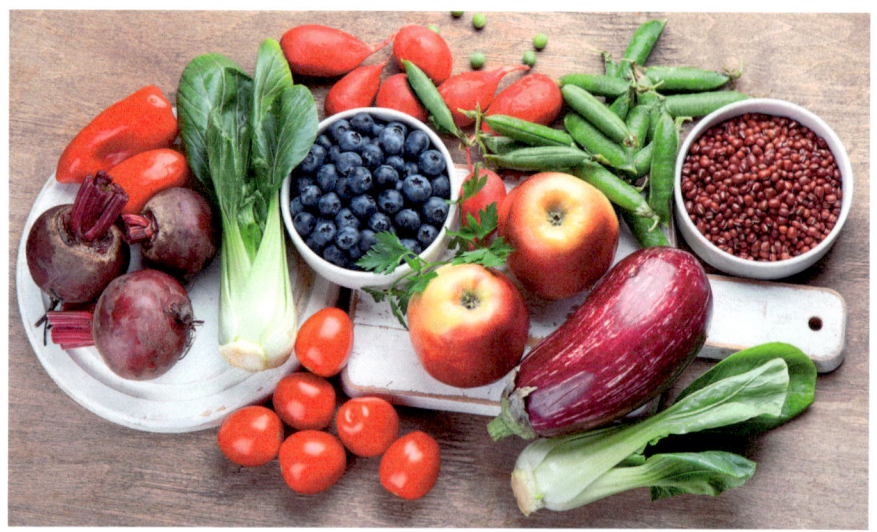

It may seem like these nutrients are adding up, and there are too many to remember. You may be feeling a bit overwhelmed, especially if some of these names are new to you. You may be thinking that it will be impossible to incorporate all thirty of these nutrients into your diet.

However, let me reassure you - it is possible to get all these in your diet, and not that difficult. Please refer to Part II of *Beyond Carrots,* "The Therapeutic Foods For Eye Health A to Z", where I put everything together.

Anti-Inflammatory

The third vital category to support healthy eyesight is the class of anti-inflammatory nutrients. Why are anti-inflammatory nutrients so critical to eye health?

Inflammation is the root cause of many chronic diseases, including vision-threatening eye disease. Let me repeat this –

Inflammation is the root cause of chronic disease.

Inflammation is a well-known underlying driver for conditions such as:

- ischemic heart disease
- stroke
- certain cancers
- diabetes mellitus
- chronic kidney disease
- autoimmune disease
- neurodegenerative conditions
- non-alcoholic fatty liver disease (NAFLD)

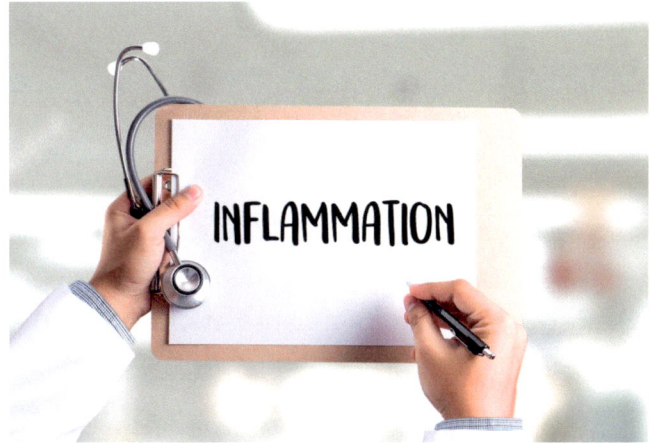

Like oxidation, as described in the section above, inflammation is part of your body's normal function and essential for survival. For example, in response to an acute stressor such as a physical injury or infection, your body will mount a reactive inflammatory reaction. Usually, this type of inflammation is transient; once the stressor is no longer present, the inflammation subsides.

However, if your body is exposed to a persistent stressor, such as chronic infection, a pro-inflammatory diet, nutrient deficiency, physical inactivity, environmental toxicants, or psychological stress, then chronic inflammation may develop. It is chronic inflammation that may predispose you to disease states.

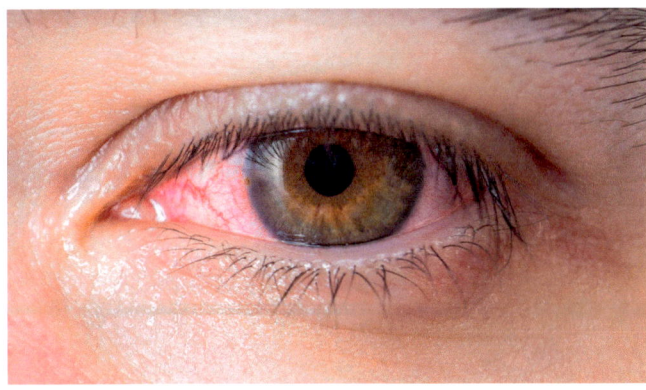

There is abundant evidence that inflammation plays a vital role as a root cause of many eye conditions, including dry eye, glaucoma, and macular degeneration.

The key to inflammatory diseases of the eye is that they must be diagnosed and treated early before any permanent damage occurs. Better yet, it is best to PREVENT inflammation.

How can you prevent or reduce chronic inflammation and thus restore a healthy balance in your body? Fortunately, the answer lies within your control, in your daily nutritional and lifestyle choices.

To illustrate how inflammation can affect your health, let us take the example of a condition called "leaky gut" syndrome.

Leaky gut is a common diagnosis managed and treated by integrative and functional medicine providers. In traditional medicine, leaky gut is known as increased intestinal permeability.

Leaky gut is caused by inflammation within the gut lining. A variety of root causes may trigger the condition:

- pro-inflammatory foods
- chronic antibiotic use
- trauma
- physical or emotional stress

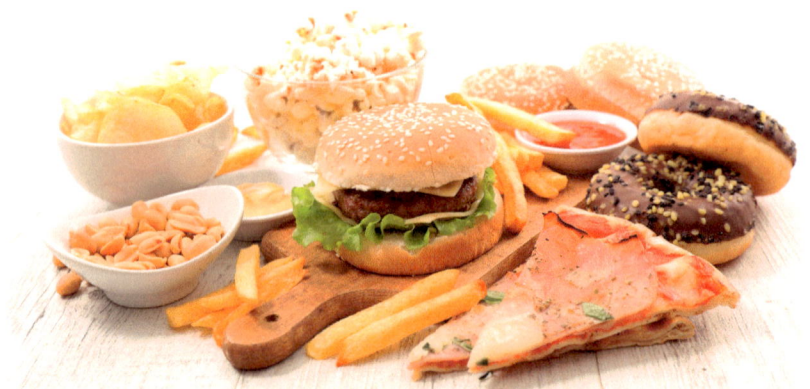

Inflammation breaks down the normal barrier within the gut lining, called tight junctions. Breakdown of the gut barrier allows individual large, undigested molecules such as gluten, a large protein found in wheat and other grain products, to penetrate the gut lining and be absorbed into the blood.

These types of large molecules are not typically exposed to the bloodstream. When recognized by surveillance immune cells within the blood, these large molecules are tagged as foreign.

In response to this foreign "invader," the body's immune system is triggered to mount an inflammatory response, thus creating more inflammation and a vicious cycle.

Leaky gut has been linked to a range of chronic inflammatory health conditions, including:

- celiac disease
- inflammatory bowel disease
    - Crohn's disease
    - ulcerative colitis
- irritable bowel syndrome (IBS)
- chronic fatigue syndrome
- fibromyalgia
- allergies
- arthritis
- asthma
- acne
- autoimmune disorders
    - lupus
    - multiple sclerosis
    - type I diabetes

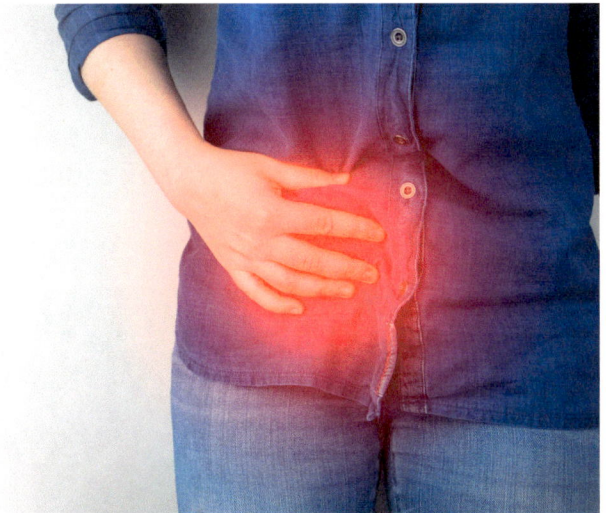

There are other types of leaky syndromes that have been described as well, such as "leaky brain," "leaky heart," and "leaky skin."

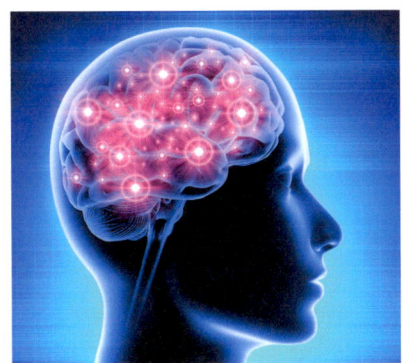
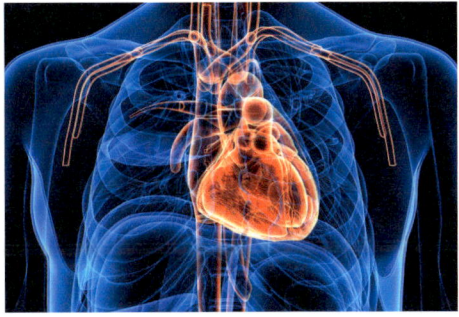
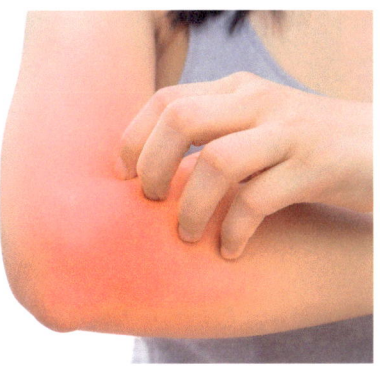

There is an analogy in the eye that I have termed "leaky eye syndrome." Leaky eye is caused by inflammation in the eye that gives rise to new blood vessels. However, these new blood vessels are not healthy and normal; they are fragile and can leak blood, proteins, and fluid. If leaky eye syndrome develops, the ultimate result is vision loss.

Similar to leaky gut, there are different causes of leaky eye syndrome. I have identified two common retinal conditions, diabetic retinopathy, and macular degeneration, as prototypical leaky eye syndromes.

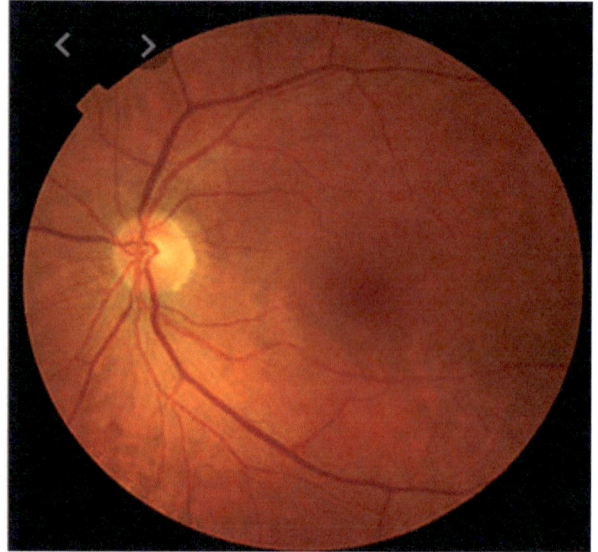

Normal healthy retina

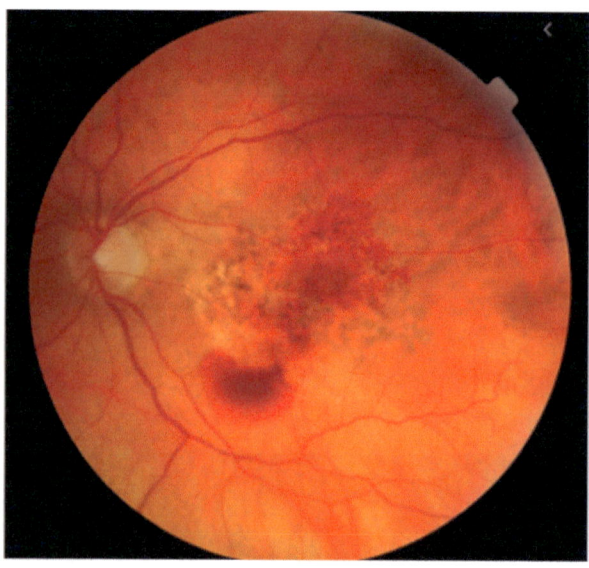

Retina with bleeding from macular degeneration, a type of "leaky eye" syndrome

There are also forms of corneal disease and inflammation in the eye (known as uveitis) that can be considered forms of leaky eye syndrome. Inflammation is the underlying cause of all these types of leaky eye syndromes.

Similar to leaky gut, healthy nutrition is key to preventing or reversing many of these leaky eye syndromes.

To ensure optimal eye health and prevent inflammatory syndromes such as leaky eye, it is paramount to include anti-inflammatory foods in your diet while avoiding pro-inflammatory foods.

Below is a list of the potent anti-inflammatory nutrients that are important to protect your vision:

- Alpha-linolenic acid (ALA, an omega-3 fatty acid)
- Eicosapentaenoic acid (EPA, an omega-3 fatty acid)
- Docosahexaenoic acid (DHA, an omega-3 fatty acid)
- Gamma-linolenic acid (GLA, an omega-6 fatty acid)
- Vitamin D
- Curcumin
- Probiotics
- Prebiotics

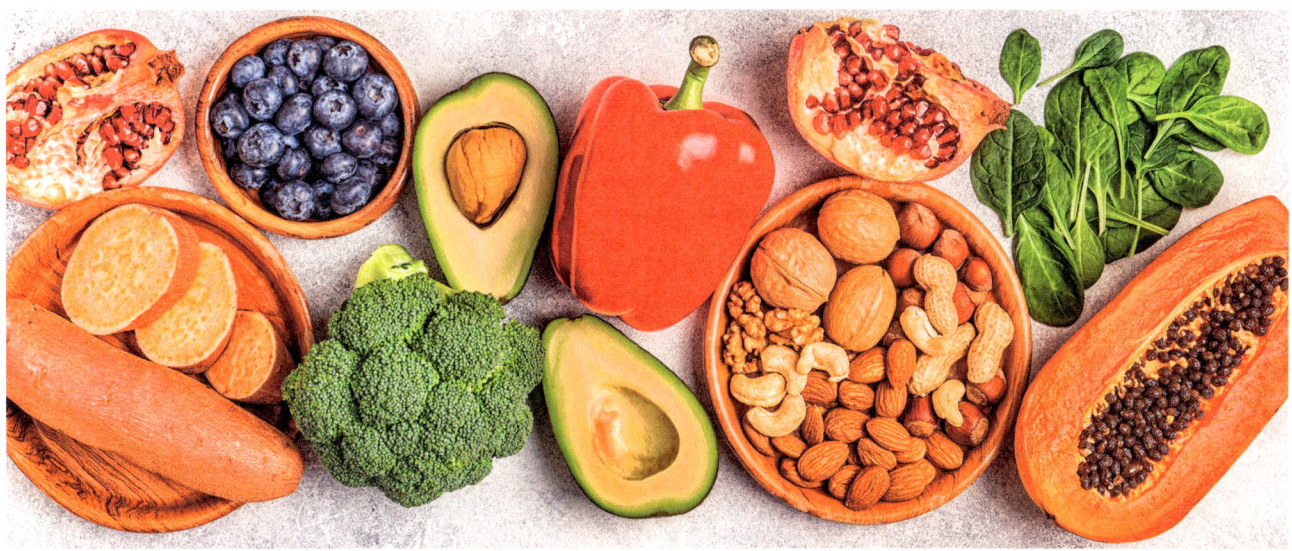

Many of the antioxidants mentioned in the previous section are also potent anti-inflammatory nutrients. Again, fortunately, there is overlap within the three major categories of nutrients needed to protect your eyesight.

To see the full list of 30+ nutrients from all three categories important for healthy vision - energy, antioxidant, and anti-inflammatory - please see the tables on the following pages.

Table 1
The 30+ Nutrients Your Eyes Need to Stay Healthy

Energy	Antioxidant	Anti-Inflammatory
Vitamin B1 (thiamine)	Vitamin A	Alpha-linolenic acid (ALA, an omega-3 fatty acid)
Vitamin B2 (riboflavin)	Vitamin C (ascorbic acid)	Eicosapentaenoic acid (EPA, an omega-3 fatty acid)
Vitamin B3 (niacin)	Vitamin E (tocopherol)	Docosahexaenoic acid (DHA, an omega-3 fatty acid)
Vitamin B5 (pantothenic acid)	Lutein (macular carotenoid)	Gamma-linolenic acid (GLA, an omega-6 fatty acid)
Vitamin B6 (Pyridoxine)	Zeaxanthin (macular carotenoid)	Vitamin D
Vitamin B7 (Biotin)	Meso-zeaxanthin (macular carotenoid)	Curcumin (bioflavonoid)
Vitamin B9 (Folate)	Astaxanthin (carotenoid)	Anthocyanins (bioflavonoids)
Coenzyme Q10 (CoQ10)	Glutathione	Probiotics
Vitamin C (ascorbic acid)	N-acetyl cysteine (NAC)	Prebiotics
Vitamin E (tocopherol)	Alpha Lipoic Acid (ALA)	
Carnitine (an amino acid)	Resveratrol (polyphenol)	

Table 1 Continued...
The 30+ Nutrients Your Eyes Need to Stay Healthy

Energy	Antioxidant
Taurine (an amino acid)	Tannins (polyphenol)
L-arginine (an amino acid)	Quercetin (bioflavonoid)
Iron (mineral)	Anthocyanins (bioflavonoids)
Zinc (a mineral)	Glucosinolates
Magnesium (mineral)	Crocin and Crocetin (bioflavonoids)
Manganese (a mineral)	Kaempferol (bioflavonoid)
Copper (mineral)	
Selenium (mineral)	
Alpha lipoic acid (ALA)	

When you compare the nutrients across the three categories, you will note that, fortunately, there is some duplication. Several nutrients, such as Vitamins C and E, and anthocyanins, serve multiple roles and provide cross-over benefits for your eye health.

The BEST way to get these 30+ nutrients in your diet is to include the nutrient-dense foods highlighted in Part II of this book, Therapeutic Foods for Eye Health A to Z. These foods are carefully chosen and curated based on their nutritional value. I call these foods "therapeutic" because each is rich in multiple nutrients your eyes need.

Beyond Carrots- 4 Simple Strategies for An Eye-Healthy Diet

Before you learn about the therapeutic foods in Part II of this book, I would like to introduce you to four overarching strategies when considering an eye-healthy nutrition plan that goes beyond carrots.

Strategy #1- A Plant-Rich Diet

Firstly, an eye-healthy diet is a "plant-rich" diet. Note that I am not using "plant-based," commonly referred to as vegan dietary choices. Instead, a plant-rich diet requires you to make plants and plant products – vegetables, fruits, and healthy fats (certain oils, nuts, and seeds) - the foundation of your diet. Adding flavorful herbs, colorful spices, and gut health boosters such as natural probiotic and prebiotic foods is also important.

Why are plants so important for your eyes? If you look back at Table 1, you will see that the majority of eye health nutrients within the three categories are derived from plants:

- energy production – B vitamins, vitamins C and E, minerals

- antioxidants – carotenoids (lutein, zeaxanthin, beta carotene), vitamins C and E, glutathione, alpha lipoic acid, and bioflavonoids

- anti-inflammatory nutrients – omega-3 fatty acids, curcumin, bioflavonoids, probiotics, and prebiotics

To fully implement a plant-rich eating style to support your eyes, you should strive to have at least *five* cups of plants per day in your diet. This may include a combination of raw and cooked foods.

Select animal products such as eggs and salmon also provide vital nutrients that may not be obtained in sufficient quantities from plants alone, such as vitamins A, B12, and D, the omega-3 fatty acids, DHA and EPA, iron, zinc, and certain amino acids.

Strategy #2- A Rainbow of 21 Colors

Each nutrient for your eyes is present in varying amounts in the therapeutic foods in Part II of this book. Therefore, rotating through these foods is critical to provide your eyes with the complete nutritional support they require.

One tip for cycling through therapeutic foods is what I like to call "the rule of 21." Most of us eat three meals a day, seven days a week, or 21 meals per week. The colors, or pigments, within foods provide vital nutrients necessary for vision. Thus, if you eat a different colored food with each meal, you will get 21 different colors each week. This diversity of colorful vegetables, fruits, and animal products throughout the week will provide your eyes with what they need.

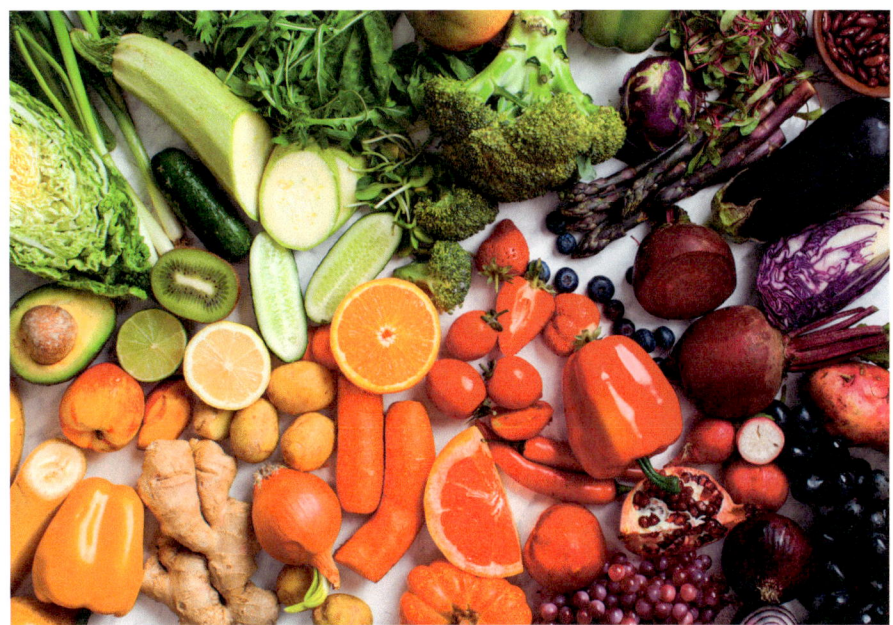

Another way to think about rotating through foods is to eat a rainbow of colors to maintain eye health. You need to eat vegetables and fruits of various shades of red, orange, yellow, green, blue, purple, black, and even white.

Remember that the rainbow you eat should come from natural foods, not colorful treats like Skittles™ or M&Ms!™

Strategy #3- Avoid 'S.A.D.' Foods

Thus far, I have shared information about which nutrients and foods are most important to support your eye health. Just as important are the foods to avoid. Many people on a Western-style diet eat foods considered 'S.A.D." foods. S.A.D. stands for Standard American Diet. This type of diet is high in:

- Unhealthy pro-inflammatory fats such as omega-6 fats (i.e., safflower and sunflower vegetable oils), saturated and trans fats (commercially prepared baked goods, potato chips, and processed meats)

- Refined and simple sugars (white bread, cereals, baked goods, soft drinks, and juices with added sugars)

- Processed foods laden with chemical preservatives (processed meats, packaged snacks)

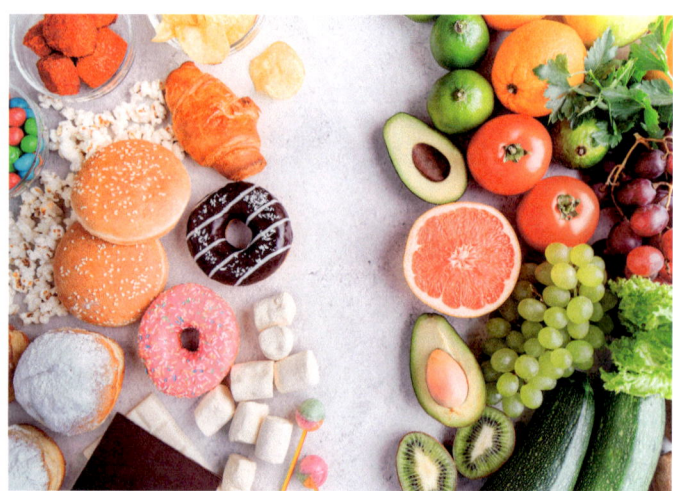

This S.A.D. style of eating increases the risk of being overweight or obese. Obesity is a pro-inflammatory state associated with many health conditions, including high blood pressure, diabetes, heart disease, and stroke, which can negatively impact your vision. Limiting S.A.D.-type foods is the best to avoid these chronic medical conditions. Instead, you should strive to eat whole, natural foods that are not processed or refined.

Strategy #4- Support Your Gut Health

You may have heard about the brain-gut connection, but have you heard about the eye-gut connection? It may sound odd that your gut health can impact your eye health. Let me explain this link between two seemingly unrelated organ systems.

An estimated 40 trillion organisms live symbiotically with you - in your gut, nostrils, oral cavity, genital tract, and brain, on your skin, and even on the surface of your eye. These organisms are your microbiome.

The organisms living within your digestive tract are collectively called the gut microbiome. The gut microbiome is an active and diverse community of bacteria, viruses, and fungi and plays a critical role in your health. These organisms help control digestion, allowing you to metabolize carbohydrates, proteins, and fats. They also interplay with your immune, nervous, endocrine, cardiovascular systems, and almost every other organ in the body, including your eyes.

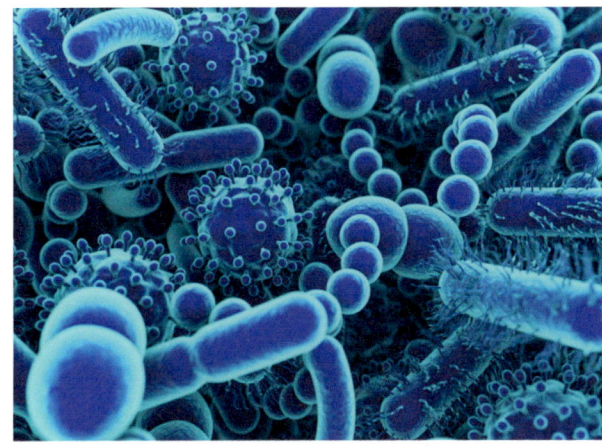

Disturbances in the gut microbiome (known as gut dysbiosis) have been linked to numerous eye conditions, such as macular degeneration, uveitis, diabetic retinopathy, dry eye (from Sjogren's syndrome), glaucoma, and infectious keratitis. Though much of this research is still in its early stages, gut dysbiosis may predispose you to inflammatory eye conditions.

The best way to support a healthy gut microbiome is to feed your gut beneficial bacteria daily to ensure that the "good" species predominate over the "bad" species. You may take probiotics as a nutritional supplement, though foods rich in live probiotics are best. The billions of live bacteria in probiotic foods like yogurt, fermented or pickled vegetables, kimchi, and sauerkraut help keep your gut healthy.

Foods known as prebiotics are also essential for a healthy gut microbiome. Prebiotics are what your gut bacteria eat to thrive. You should strive to include prebiotic foods at least 4-5 times a week into your diet to support your gut health.

Nutrients and Foods for Specific Eye Conditions

Perhaps the most common question my patients ask me is, "Dr. Banik; I have a diagnosis of … Which food should I eat?" Unfortunately, the answer is not straightforward. First, no single food can treat or cure any specific eye condition.

Despite its small size, the eye is a complex organ with over 40 parts that work together, not independently. Thus, you need the full range of nutrients and foods to support your overall eye health; there is no single magic pill, be it a nutrient or food, for vision.

That being said, if you are experiencing a specific eye issue, depending on the diagnosis and part of the eye affected, specific nutrients from particular foods may be helpful. So that you can better understand all these concepts, I'll first share an overview of eye anatomy and function. Then I will highlight specific structures of the eye and nutrients that may help address disease or dysfunction.

How does the eye work?

The eye functions similarly to a camera with film. The cornea (lens of the camera) allows light rays to enter through the pupil, the circular dark opening in the middle of the eye (the camera's aperture).

The iris, or the colored part of the eye (shutter), continuously adjusts its size to let varying amounts of light through the pupil. Next, the eye's lens, which sits behind the iris, focuses these light rays onto the back of the eye, called the retina (film of the camera).

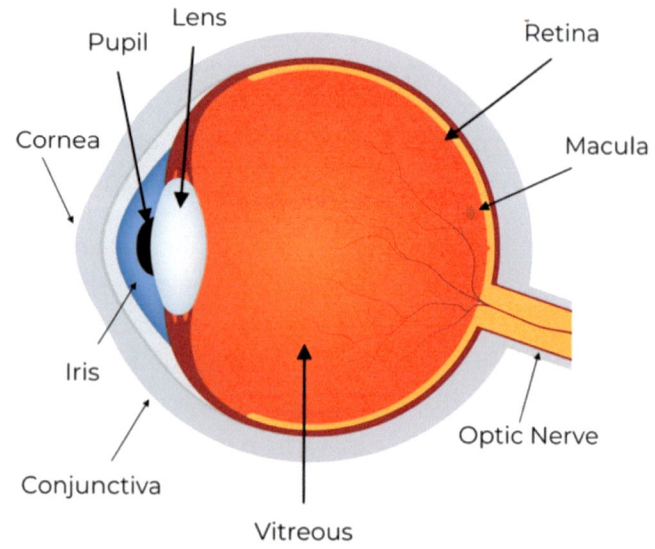

The retina captures light energy and processes it into electrical energy. The optic nerve contains over one million nerve fibers and functions like a cable, transmitting this electrical energy to the brain. The brain then processes this information to create the images you see.

The following table summarizes the essential structures of your eye, their functions, the nutrients and dietary styles that best support them, and the conditions that commonly affect the particular structure.

For more in-depth explanations, please download the bonus pdf entitled "Eye Anatomy 101" from my website, www.rudranibanikmd.com/beyondcarrots.

Table 2
Eye Structure, Function, Nutrients, and Diseases

Structure	Function	Nutrients	Diseases

conjunctiva	- transparent membrane that covers the surface of the eye and acts as a protective barrier
	- contains blood vessels and immune cells
	- contains goblet cells that secrete mucin to help lubricate the ocular surface
	- houses the ocular surface microbiome, a collection of organisms that lives on the surface of the eye
		- antioxidants
		   ◦ vitamins A, C, E
		- adequate hydration
			- damage from the sun's UV rays, wind, dust
			   ◦ pinguecula
			   ◦ pterygium
			- conjunctivitis
			   ◦ bacterial
			   ◦ viral
			   ◦ allergic
			- scarring
			   ◦ (i.e., autoimmune pemphigoid)

tear film	- coats and lubricates the ocular surface, the conjunctiva and cornea
	- derived from lacrimal glands, meibomian glands, and goblet cells
	- provides nutrients to the ocular surface
	- washes away debris
		- omega-3 fatty acids- DHA, EPA, ALA
		- omega-6 fatty acid- GLA
		- minerals
		   ◦ sodium
		   ◦ potassium
		   ◦ magnesium
		   ◦ calcium
		- hydration
		- bioflavonoids
		   ◦ curcumin
			- dry eye syndrome (DES)
			   ◦ evaporative dry eye (meibomian gland dysfunction or MGD)
			   ◦ aqueous deficiency
			      ▪ autoimmune disease (i.e., Sjogren's syndrome)

cornea	- transparent, dome-shaped, curved structure at the front of the eye
	- made out of different types of collagen
	- enables light rays to enter the eye
	- focuses light rays through the pupil and lens onto the retina at the back of the eye
		- antioxidants
		   ◦ vitamins A, C, E
		   ◦ glutathione
		   ◦ N-acetylcysteine (NAC)
		- vitamin C to support collagen production
		- vitamin B2 (riboflavin) (for certain corneal degenerations)
		- omega-3 fatty acids- DHA, EPA, ALA
			- dry eye syndrome (see categories under tear film above)
			- infections
			   ◦ keratitis
			   ◦ ulcers
			- scarring
			- degenerations & dystrophies
			   ◦ keratoconus

Table 2 Continued...
Eye Structure, Function, Nutrients, and Diseases

Structure	Function	Nutrients	Diseases
trabecular meshwork (TM)	<ul><li>drains fluid from the front of the eye</li><li>when dysfunctional or blocked, eye pressure builds up, causing damage to the optic nerve known as glaucoma</li></ul>	<ul><li>polyphenols<ul><li>bioflavonoids<ul><li>quercetin</li><li>anthocyanins</li></ul></li><li>resveratrol</li><li>curcumin</li></ul></li><li>sulforaphane</li><li>antioxidants<ul><li>vitamins A, C, E</li><li>glutathione</li><li>N-acetylcysteine (NAC)</li></ul></li><li>omega-3 fatty acids<ul><li>DHA, EPA, ALA</li></ul></li></ul>	<ul><li>glaucoma<ul><li>open angle</li><li>closed angle</li></ul></li><li>trauma</li><li>infection<ul><li>herpes</li></ul></li></ul>
iris	<ul><li>colored (pigmented) part of the eye</li><li>dynamic structure, changes shape to allow light to enter eye through its opening, the pupil</li></ul>	<ul><li>polyphenols<ul><li>bioflavonoids</li></ul></li><li>antioxidants<ul><li>vitamins A, C, E</li><li>glutathione</li><li>N-acetylcysteine (NAC)</li></ul></li></ul>	<ul><li>inflammation<ul><li>uveitis</li></ul></li><li>glaucoma</li><li>infection<ul><li>herpes</li></ul></li><li>trauma</li><li>tumors<ul><li>melanoma</li><li>metastasis</li></ul></li><li>scarring</li></ul>
lens	<ul><li>clear structure suspended behind the iris, the colored part of the eye</li><li>focuses light rays that have entered the eye through the cornea and pupil onto the retina</li></ul>	<ul><li>antioxidants<ul><li>vitamins A, C, E</li><li>glutathione</li></ul></li><li>macular carotenoids<ul><li>lutein</li><li>zeaxanthin</li></ul></li><li>for diabetics and pre-diabetics, low glycemic index foods</li></ul>	<ul><li>cataract (opacity of the lens) due to oxidative damage from UV light and metabolic stress<ul><li>age-related</li><li>diabetic</li><li>traumatic</li><li>radiation damage</li></ul></li><li>lens dislocation<ul><li>trauma</li><li>pseudoexfoliation syndrome</li></ul></li></ul>

Table 2 Continued...
Eye Structure, Function, Nutrients, and Diseases

Structure	Function	Nutrients	Diseases
retina	<ul><li>light-sensing tissue at the back of the eye</li><li>has 9 layers of cells</li><li>retinal photoreceptors capture and process wavelengths of light and convert light energy into electrical energy</li><li>high metabolic rate, needs lots of energy to function well</li><li>creates many waste by-products</li></ul>	<ul><li>macular carotenoids<ul><li>lutein</li><li>zeaxanthin</li><li>meso-zeaxanthin</li></ul></li><li>astaxanthin</li><li>antioxidants<ul><li>glutathione</li><li>vitamins C and E</li></ul></li><li>minerals<ul><li>copper</li><li>selenium</li><li>zinc</li><li>iron</li></ul></li><li>B vitamins</li><li>Vitamin A (for light processing)</li><li>omega-3s<ul><li>DHA, EPA</li></ul></li><li>low glycemic diet</li></ul>	<ul><li>macular degeneration</li><li>diabetic retinopathy</li><li>hypertensive retinopathy</li><li>retinal stroke<ul><li>arterial occlusion</li><li>venous occlusion</li></ul></li><li>retinal tear or detachment</li><li>vitamin A deficiency</li><li>infectious retinitis<ul><li>HIV</li><li>syphilis</li><li>herpes and other viruses</li><li>bacteria</li><li>parasites</li><li>fungi</li></ul></li><li>inflammation<ul><li>white dot syndromes (may also affect underlying choroid)</li></ul></li></ul>
optic nerve	<ul><li>connects the eye to the brain via axons of retinal ganglion cells</li><li>each optic nerve contains over 1.2 million axons that transmit electrical signals</li><li>has high energy demands and a high metabolic rate</li></ul>	<ul><li>B vitamins<ul><li>cobalamin (B12)</li><li>folate (B9)</li></ul></li><li>antioxidants<ul><li>glutathione</li><li>vitamins C and E</li></ul></li><li>minerals<ul><li>copper, selenium, zinc, iron</li></ul></li><li>bioflavonoids<ul><li>resveratrol</li></ul></li><li>Vitamin D</li><li>omega-3s<ul><li>DHA, EPA</li></ul></li><li>curcumin</li></ul>	<ul><li>glaucoma</li><li>inflammation<ul><li>optic neuritis</li><li>perineuritis</li></ul></li><li>optic nerve stroke</li><li>swelling of the optic nerve from high pressure in the brain (aka "papilledema")</li><li>diabetic papillitis</li><li>optic neuropathies<ul><li>hereditary</li><li>toxic</li><li>metabolic</li></ul></li></ul>

To make it easier for you to identify which foods in Part II have the nutrients needed to support different parts of the eye, I have listed categories of eye conditions that may benefit under the therapeutic foods. The four categories are designated by the letters:

C - Cornea, Conjunctiva, and Tear Film
L - Lens
O - Optic Nerve and Trabecular Meshwork
R - Retina

As you go through the therapeutic foods, you will see much overlap in the nutrients they contain and which eye conditions these nutrients may benefit. For example, leafy greens and berries are rich sources of vitamins A and C, two essential antioxidants in the fight against dry eye, cataracts, and macular degeneration.

This duplication is intentional, as it is best to have multiple sources of crucial nutrients and rotate through these foods during the week to provide your eyes with the full spectrum they need to remain healthy.

Beyond nutrition, remember that many other factors determine your eye health status - genetics, age, sex, eye and skin pigmentation, UV exposure, body weight, composition, activity level, environment, toxins, and stressors. These topics are beyond the scope of nutrition and would require an additional book to discuss!

To help you determine which eye structures you should support through specific nutrients and foods, I encourage you to take a free online assessment called the Nutrition Eye-Q Test. I developed this unique tool in conjunction with this book to help you personalize your ocular nutrition.

By answering simple questions about your medical and eye history, current diet, and lifestyle habits, you will receive a personalized report. This report will highlight which nutrients and foods you should focus on based on the 4 categories noted above- C, L, O, and R. Your Nutrition Eye-Q results will serve as your guide to the foods in Part II of this book, so you can keep your eyes healthy and eat right for your sight!

To take the online Nutrition Eye-Q Test, simply scan this QR code with your smartphone camera-

Summary

Nutrition is the cornerstone of preventing eye disease, and many foods beyond carrots are necessary to provide your eyes with the many nutrients they need to stay healthy.

Your eyes are complex organs that use a great deal of energy and are susceptible to oxidative damage and inflammation. To fight against these stressors and safeguard your vision, an eye-healthy diet including over 30 crucial nutrients is necessary.

This eye-healthy diet will supply your cells with the vitamins and minerals required to function effectively and protect against cellular damage. Nutritious food will strengthen your body's immune system, support your gut microbiome, and help keep inflammation at bay. If you eat right, you are working to protect your sight.

Remember: Food is Medicine.

Another famous adage to keep in mind when it comes to eye health is this:

An ounce of prevention is worth a pound of cure.

Healthy nutritional habits must be started early, even in childhood, long before many age-related eye diseases, such as cataracts, glaucoma, and macular degeneration, settle in. Many eye diseases are not reversible, and thus it is best to prevent them rather than treat them after they develop.

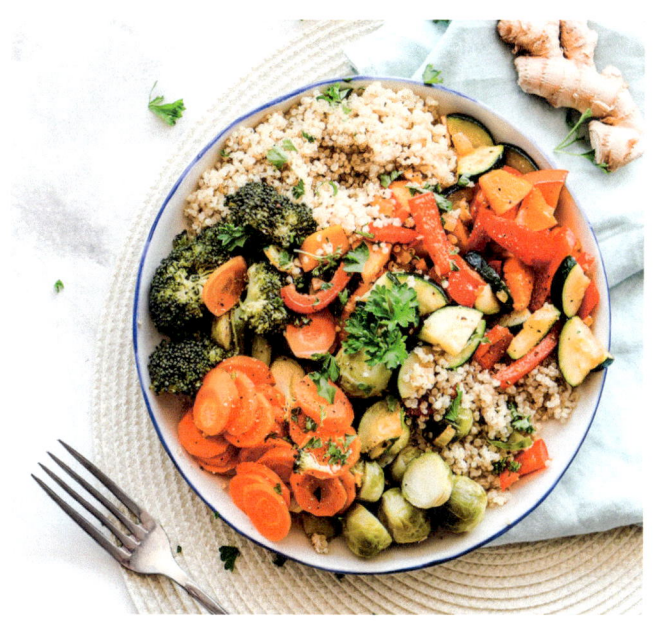

Finally, the most important thing to remember about preventing eye disease is that these strategies are under your control. You can choose your nutrition; you have the power to make healthy choices over unhealthy ones. It is now time to begin exercising your power.

Let's now take a journey through the foods richest in the 30+ nutrients you need for your eyes, those I have curated as the best foods for eye health, A to Z.

Part II

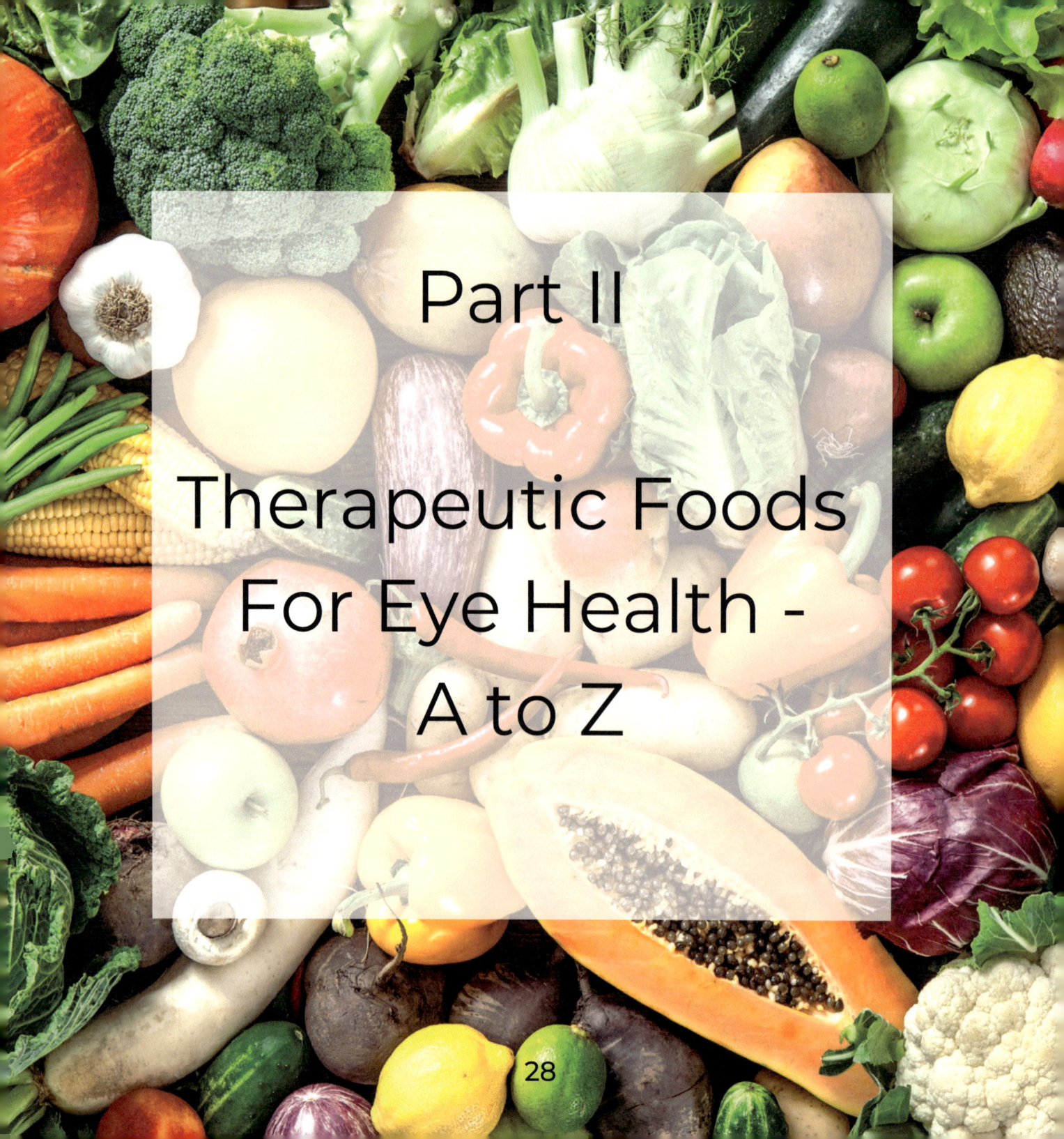

Therapeutic Foods For Eye Health - A to Z

A

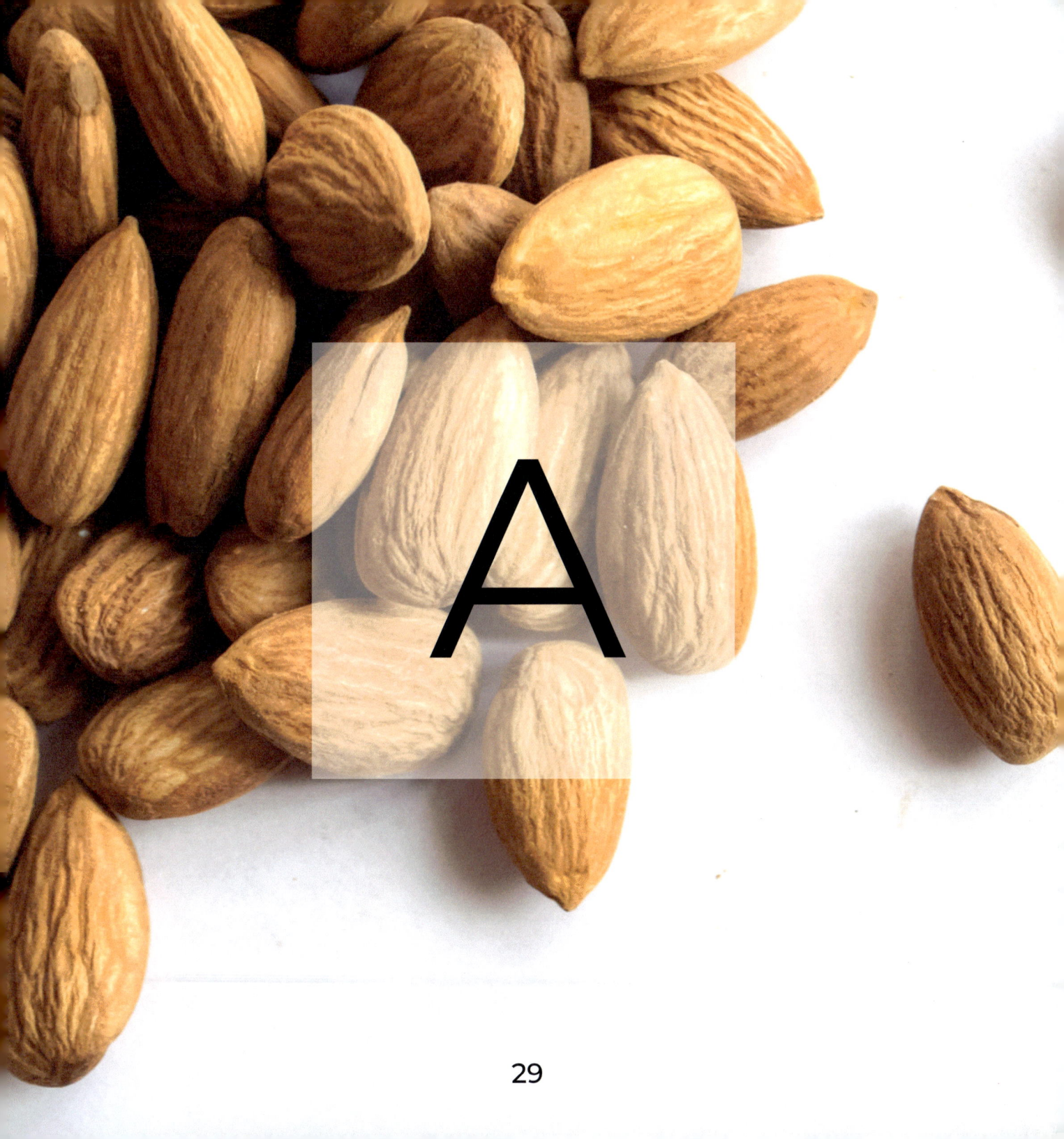

almonds

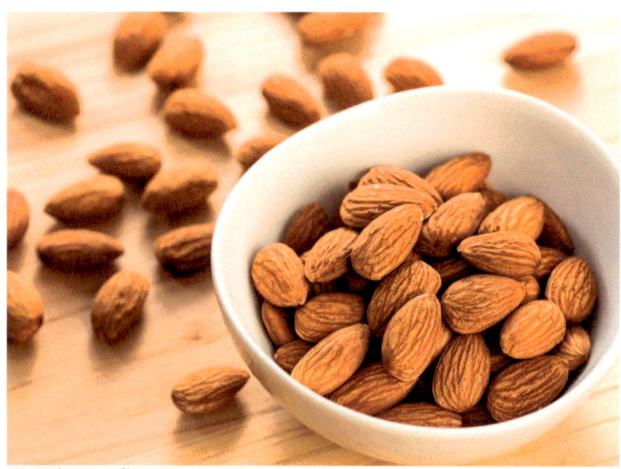

Almonds are tree nuts packed with antioxidants such as polyphenols (found in their brown skin) and vitamin E. These antioxidants can help protect against age-related eye diseases like cataracts, macular degeneration, and glaucoma.

Almonds are an excellent source of magnesium, a mineral essential to help regulate blood sugar, insulin levels, and blood pressure. Almonds are also a good source of riboflavin (Vitamin B2), a key nutrient to support energy production for the eye's high metabolic demands.

Eye benefits: C, L, O, R

Almonds have been shown to help lower cholesterol and modulate weight, both important for eye health. Finally, almonds are high in fiber, helping to promote gut health via digestion and detoxification.

avocado

Avocado is a fruit considered a superfood for eye and brain health. Avocado is rich in the antioxidants that support retinal health, such as lutein, zeaxanthin, and vitamin E, all essential to prevent age-related macular degeneration.

Avocado is packed with key B vitamins critical for efficient energy metabolism - B1, B2, and B3. Avocado is also high in healthy monounsaturated fats, which aid in absorbing fat-soluble vitamins. Finally, avocado has been shown to help lower bad cholesterol, lowering the risk for strokes that may affect vision.

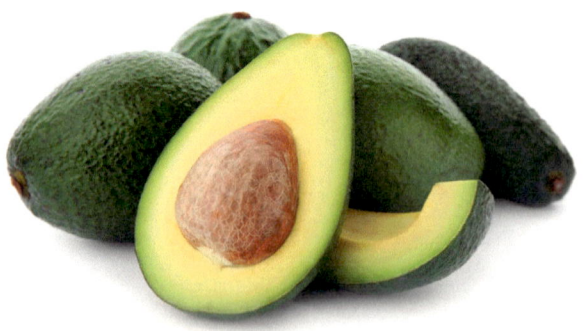

Eye benefits: O, R

B

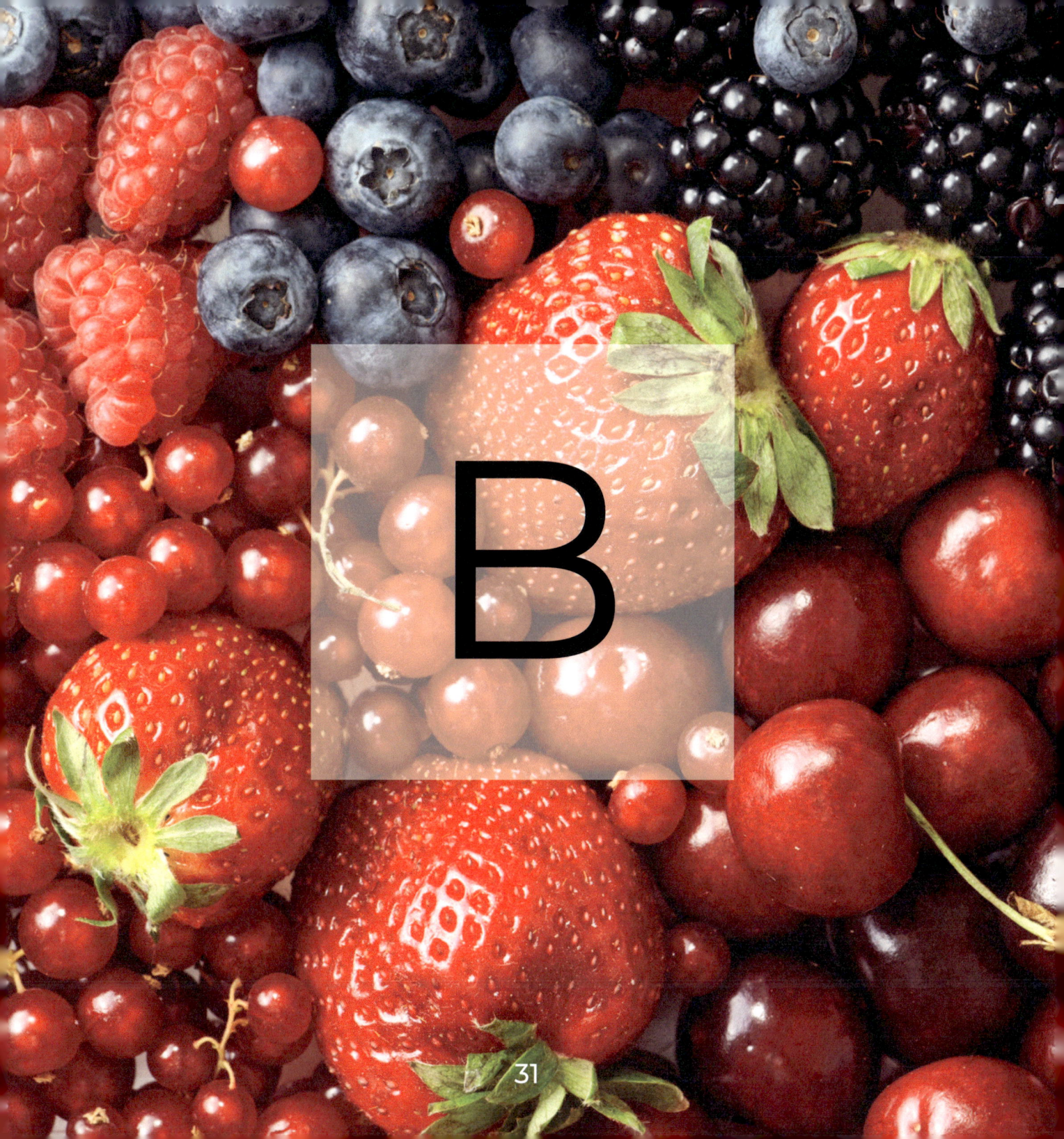

bell peppers

Bell peppers are fruits that come from the *Capsicum* plant. They belong to the nightshade family and are related to other nightshades like tomatoes and chili peppers. When harvested early, bell peppers are green; they may turn bright red in color when ripened. In addition, some varieties come in orange, yellow, and purple.

Bell peppers contain many vital nutrients for eye health. Firstly, they are an excellent source of vitamin C, essential for antioxidant protection, structural support, and immune health.

Bell peppers, particularly the orange and yellow varieties, also provide high amounts of lutein and zeaxanthin, two carotenoids located at the macula at the retina's center. These carotenoids serve as the eye's UV and blue-blocking filters, like built-in sunglasses. Bell peppers also contain beta carotene, a carotenoid that can be converted to vitamin A. Adequate vitamin A is necessary to prevent night blindness and dry eye.

Bell peppers also provide a variety of antioxidant compounds, including lycopene, capsanthin, violaxanthin, quercetin, and luteolin. These powerful pigmented nutrients are best released when the fruit is heated and cooked in olive oil. Finally, bell peppers provide fiber, essential for healthy digestion and the gut microbiome.

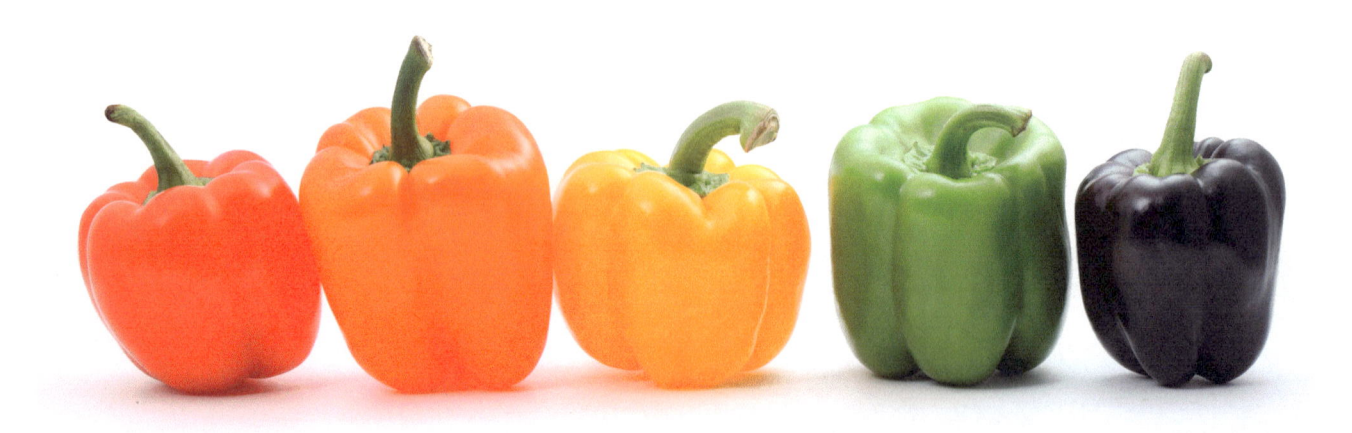

Eye benefits: C, L, O, R

berries

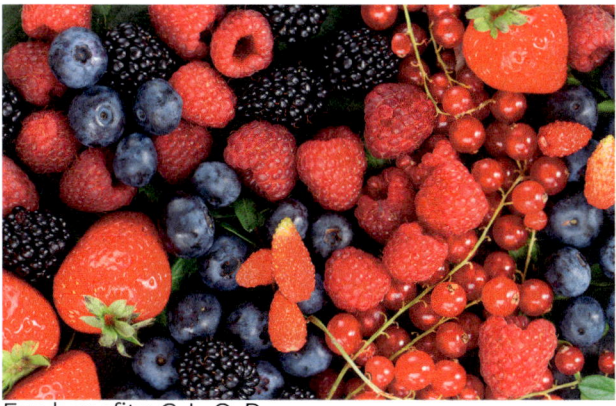

Eye benefits: C, L, O, R

All berries, including acai, blackberry, blueberry, goji berry, raspberry, and strawberry, provide many eye-healthy nutrients. All berries are packed with anthocyanins. These pigments give these fruits their vibrant color and serve as potent antioxidants. Anthocyanins improve blood flow and protect against free radical damage in the eye and brain. Strawberries and dark-blue or purplish berries, such as blueberries and blackberries, have been shown to improve memory and cognition.

Berries also provide:
- Vitamin C to protect against free radical damage, and support collagen formation in the eye
- Vitamin A to prevent night blindness and fight dry eye
- Vitamin E to protect against free radical damage and oxidative stress
- Quercetin, a flavonoid, to serve as an antioxidant

Berries have a low glycemic impact, decreasing the risk of spikes in blood sugar and damage to the eye from diabetes. Berries are an excellent fiber source, helping promote gut health.

Brazil nuts

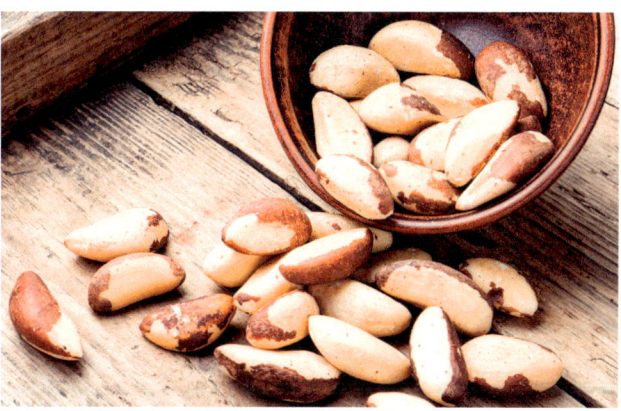

In general, nuts are essential for eye health because they provide antioxidants such as glutathione and vitamin E, with Brazil nuts providing additional unique benefits. Brazil nuts contain high concentrations of selenium, a mineral critical for healthy metabolism and efficient energy production. Selenium is also vital for thyroid function and has improved the symptoms and signs of thyroid eye disease. This autoimmune condition may develop associated with Hashimoto's thyroiditis or Graves' disease.

Eye benefits: C, L, O

C

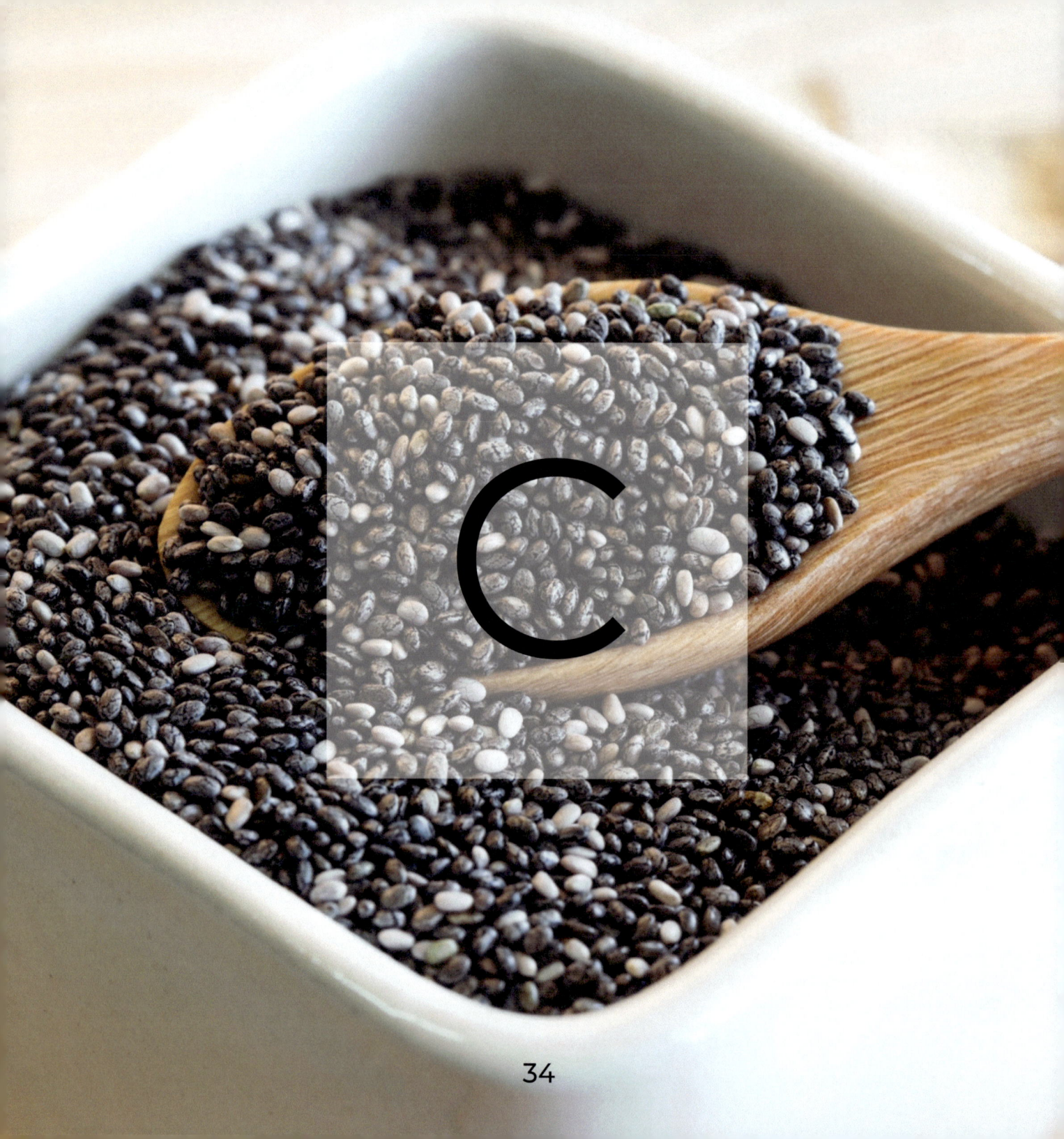

cherries

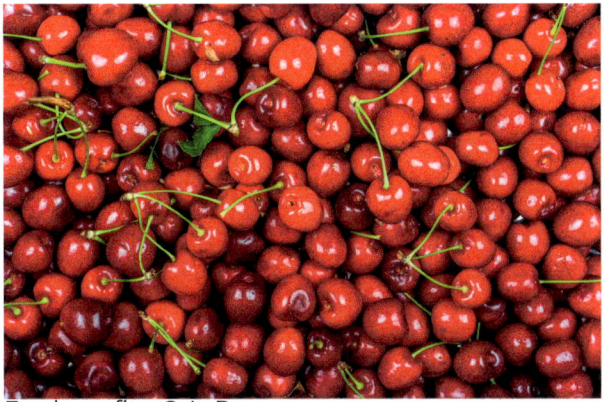

Eye benefits: C, L, R

Cherries contain potent antioxidant and anti-inflammatory compounds called polyphenols that fight against oxidative stress and inflammation. Polyphenol-rich diets have been shown to protect against many chronic conditions, including heart disease and diabetes, and thus are indirectly beneficial for eye health.

Cherries also have vitamin C and carotenoids such as beta carotene that may protect against free radicals and oxidative damage that are the root causes of age-related eye diseases such as cataracts, glaucoma, and macular degeneration. Cherries have. a low glycemic index, limiting blood sugar spikes and diabetic complications. Cherries are also an excellent source of fiber, thus helpful in promoting gut health.

chia seeds

Despite their tiny size, chia seeds are packed with essential nutrients for eye health. Chia seeds are high in alpha-linolenic acid (ALA). The body converts ALA into DHA and EPA. These three omega-3 fatty acids are anti-inflammatory and support a healthy ocular surface to prevent dry eye. Omega-3s have been associated with a reduced risk for vision loss from macular degeneration. Chia seeds are an excellent source of vitamins and minerals essential for the eye's energy production, including thiamine (B1), niacin (B3), magnesium, iron, and zinc. A single serving of 2 tablespoons of chia seeds contains almost 10 grams of fiber, which is wonderful for promoting gut health.

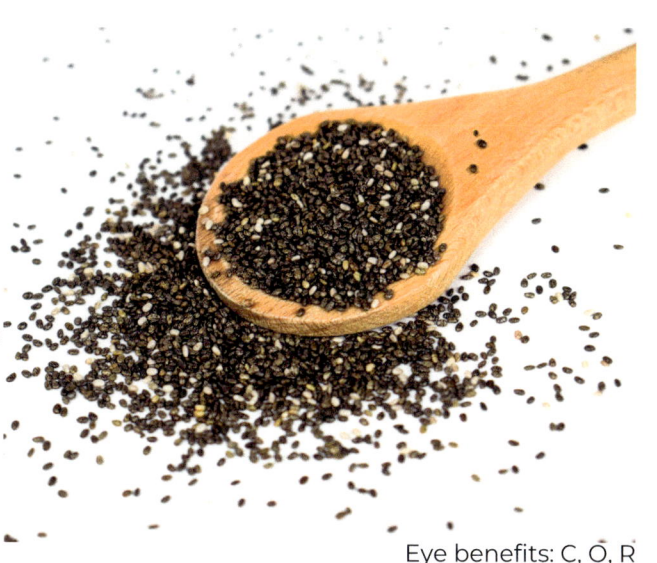

Eye benefits: C, O, R

cruciferous vegetables

Cruciferous vegetables (also known as Brassicas) are anti-inflammatory and promote detoxification. Research has shown that crucifers act as powerful antioxidants, stimulate the immune system, and slow cognitive decline.

Crucifers contain a key compound called sulforaphane. Sulforaphane helps protect the body from excessive inflammation by ramping up the production of glutathione, the body's internal antioxidant. Glutathione is key to fighting against oxidative damage and protecting against age-related eye conditions such as cataracts, glaucoma, and macular degeneration.

The best cruciferous vegetables for eye health include:

-Broccoli
-Broccoli sprouts
-Broccoli rabe
-Cauliflower
-Cabbage
-Brussels sprouts
-Turnips
-Kohlrabi
-Radishes
-Daikon radishes
-Leafy greens - kale, collard greens, and mustard greens, arugula, watercress, bok choy

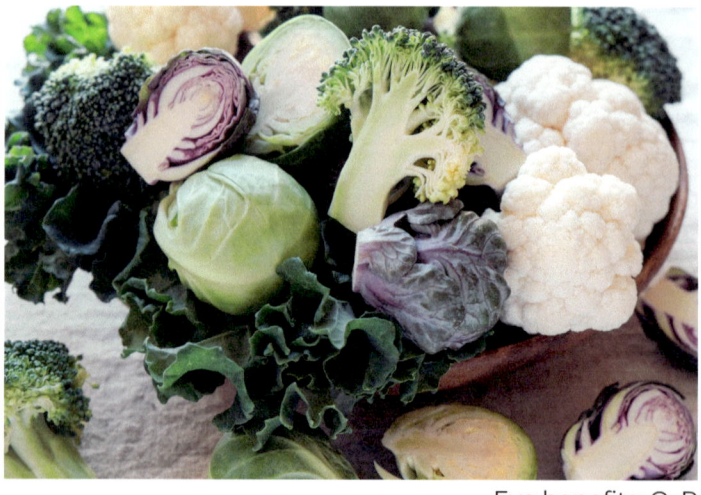

Eye benefits: O, R

Cruciferous vegetables are also associated with many other health benefits. They are associated with a reduced risk of heart disease and many cancers. Long-term studies have correlated eating vegetables in the broccoli family with longevity.

Also, many cruciferous vegetables are good plant-based sources of protein. For example, broccoli contains 5 grams of protein per 1 cup serving!

D

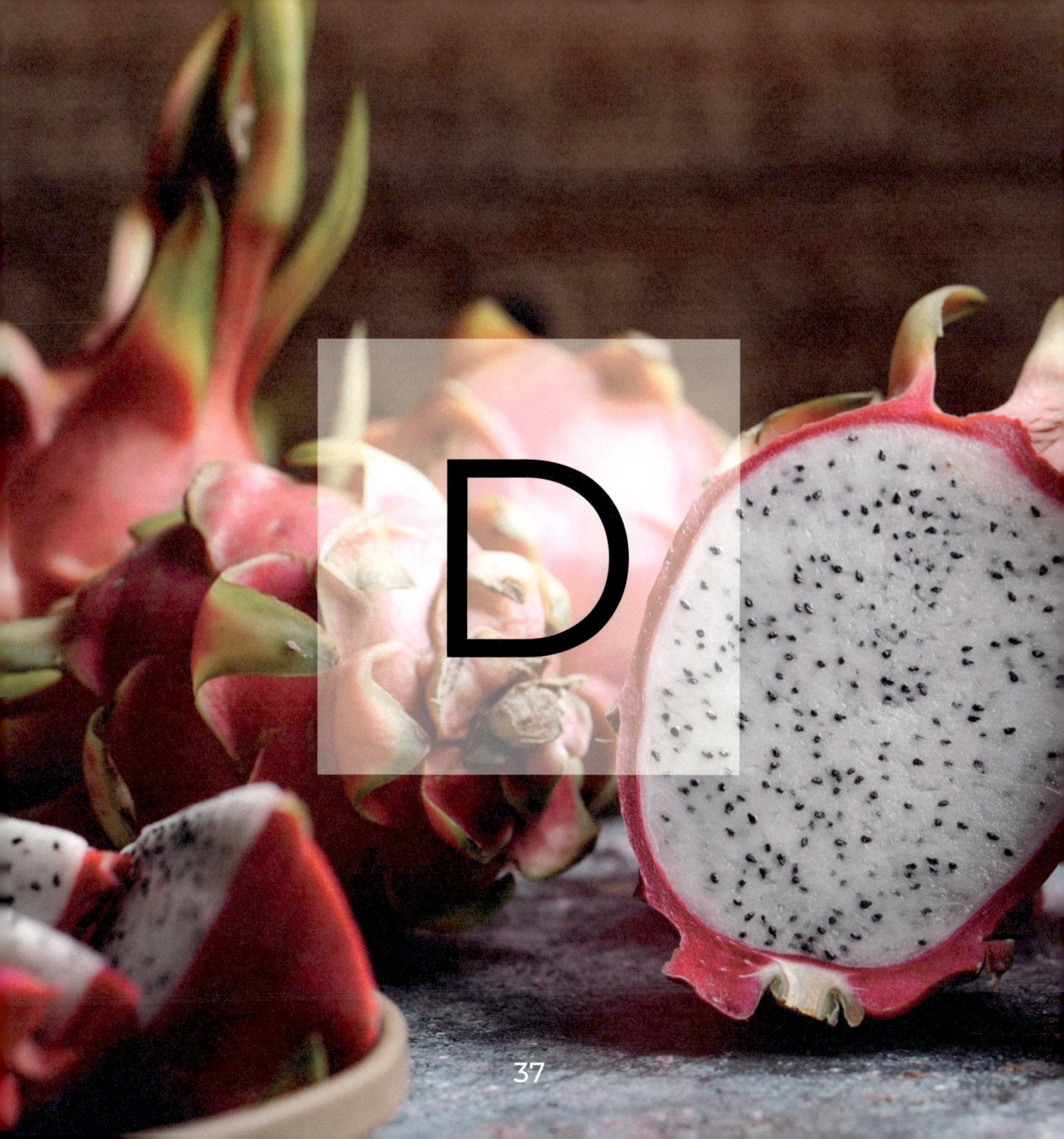

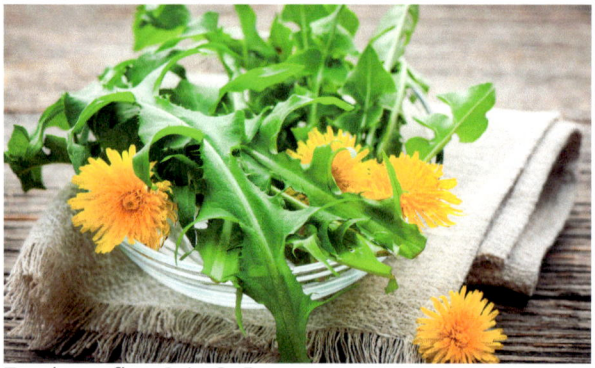

dandelion greens

Though often considered an undesirable weed, the dandelion plant has many health benefits. All its parts – the roots, stem, leaves, and flower - can be consumed. When it comes to eye health, dandelion greens are incredibly nutrient-rich. They are packed with lutein and zeaxanthin, two macular pigments that serve as our eyes' internal sunglasses and blue blockers. Consuming dandelion greens may help lower your risk of developing macular degeneration and cataracts.

Eye benefits: C, L, O, R

Dandelion greens provide many other essential vitamins, minerals, and polyphenols, such as Vitamin A, C, E, K, folate, iron, magnesium, and potassium. Here's a quick tip about dandelion greens – they are bitter, so they are best lightly boiled, sauteed with garlic or olive oil, or added to a green smoothie. Dandelion tea also has potent detoxifying properties.

dragonfruit

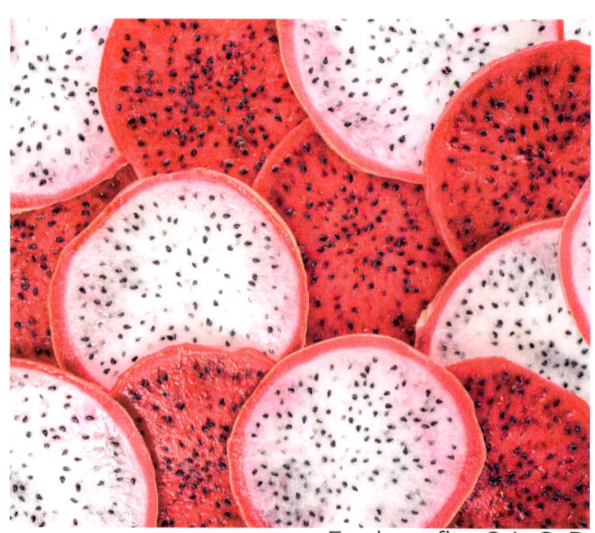

Dragon fruit, also called strawberry pear or pitaya, catches the eye with its vibrant, crimson skin and seed-speckled pulp. Dragon fruit provides Vitamin C and beta carotene (a precursor to Vitamin A), both strong antioxidant compounds that fight oxidative stress. Dragon fruit also contains betalains and lycopene, plant-derived antioxidant compounds. Together, these vitamins and nutrients may help fight age-related conditions such as cataracts and macular degeneration. Dragon fruit is an excellent source of magnesium and iron, both important for energy production and metabolism. Finally, dragon fruit is an excellent source of prebiotics and fiber, helping to support your gut microbiome.

Eye benefits: C, L, O, R

extra virgin olive oil

Eye benefits: C, L, O, R

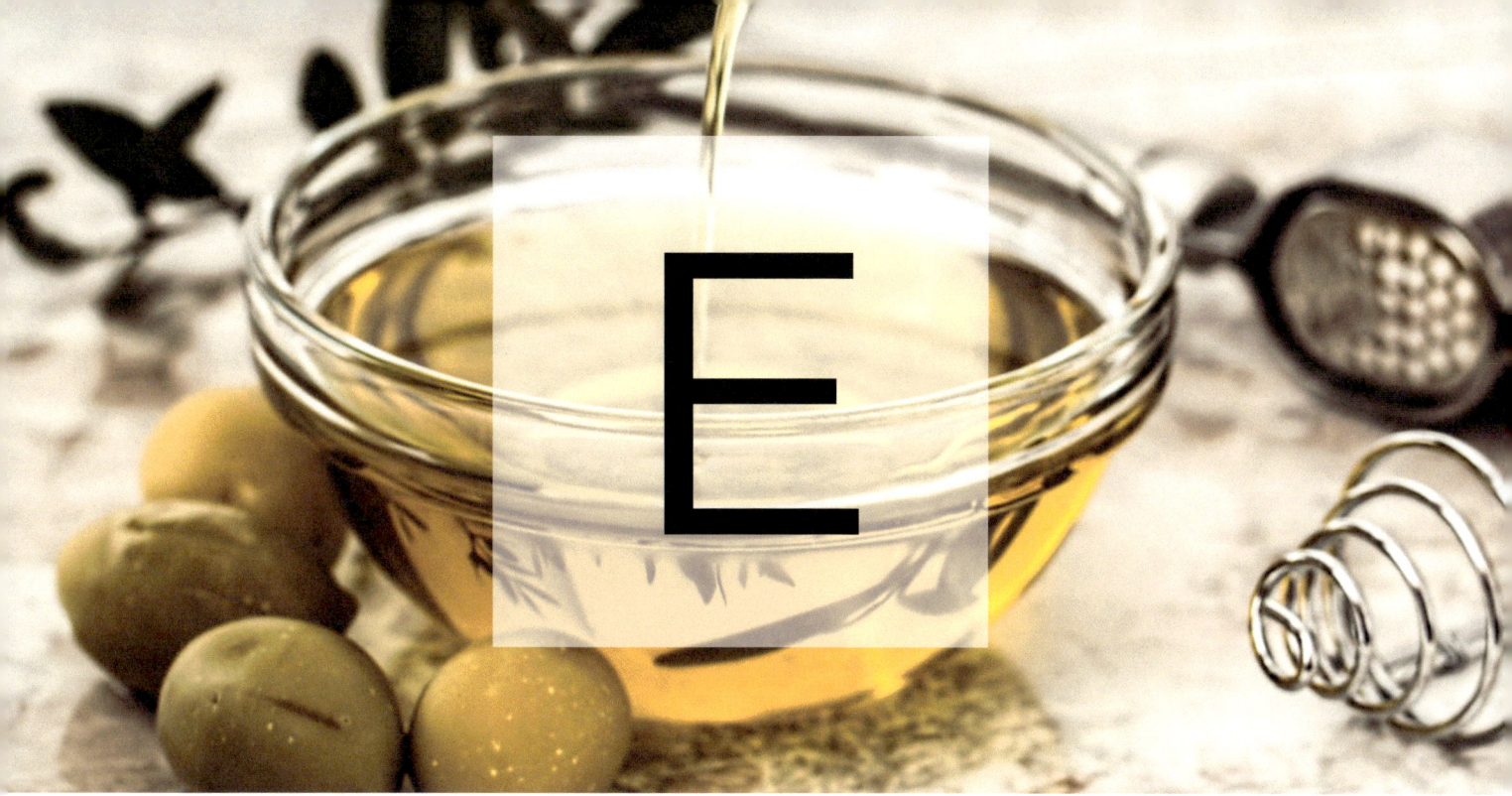

Many would argue that olive oil is nature's healthiest fat. Olive oil has been used for millennia as a staple in the Mediterranean diet and has been proven to have heart, cholesterol, brain, and anti-inflammatory benefits.

Olive oil contains several different types of fat, with monounsaturated oleic acid being the predominant type. Oleic acid is an omega-9 fatty acid that is anti-inflammatory. Olive oil also provides smaller amounts of polyunsaturated essential omega-3 and omega-6 fatty acids.

In addition, as proven in numerous clinical studies, olive oil contains vitamins E and K, as well as powerful polyphenol antioxidants that reduce the risk of chronic disease. Research has also shown that olive oil helps combat diabetes type 2, heart disease, and stroke; all three should be avoided to maintain excellent vision and brain health.

Due to its high concentration of monounsaturated fat, olive oil can be used in a variety of cooking at high temperatures. Always choose extra virgin olive oil (EVOO) to ensure the highest concentration of nutrients without dilution.

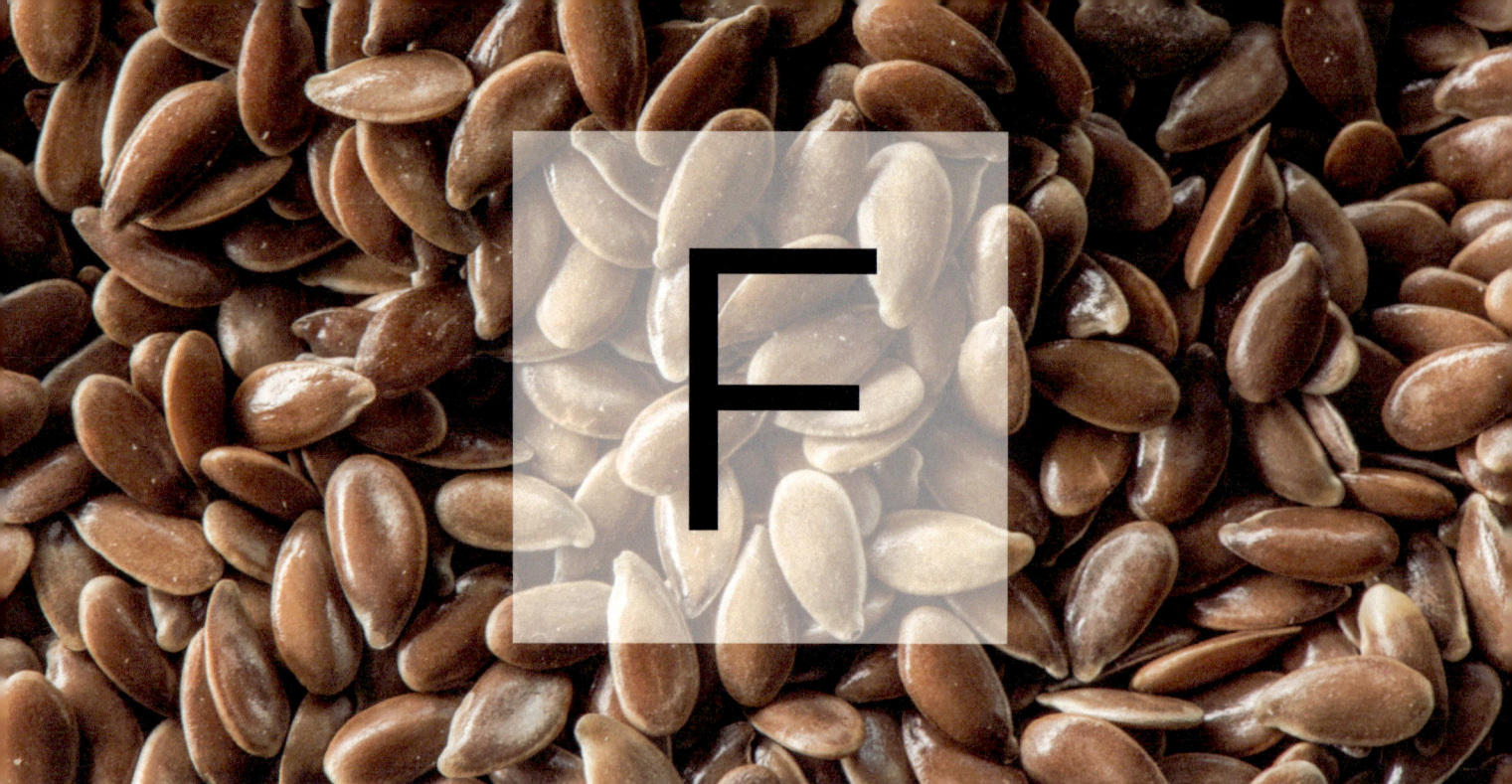

Eye benefits: C, R

flax seeds

Flax seeds have been cultivated since the beginnings of agricultural civilization. They are packed with macronutrients; just one tablespoon provides quality healthy fats, protein, and fiber.

Flax seeds are an excellent plant-based source of an essential omega-3 fatty acid, alpha-linolenic acid (ALA). ALA is anti-inflammatory. The body can convert ALA into two other essential healthy omega-3 fats, DHA and EPA. DHA is vital for eye health since the highest concentration of DHA in the body is found in the cell membranes of retinal photoreceptors. These cells have a high metabolic rate with constant turnover. Their cell membranes need to be replenished with DHA. DHA and EPA have also proven helpful in the fight against macular degeneration and dry eye. Flaxseed oil is higher in ALA than ground flax seeds.

Flax seeds are beneficial in regulating cholesterol, blood pressure, and blood sugar, all important for maintaining eye health. Flax seeds also have both soluble and insoluble fiber that helps maintain your gut health.

G

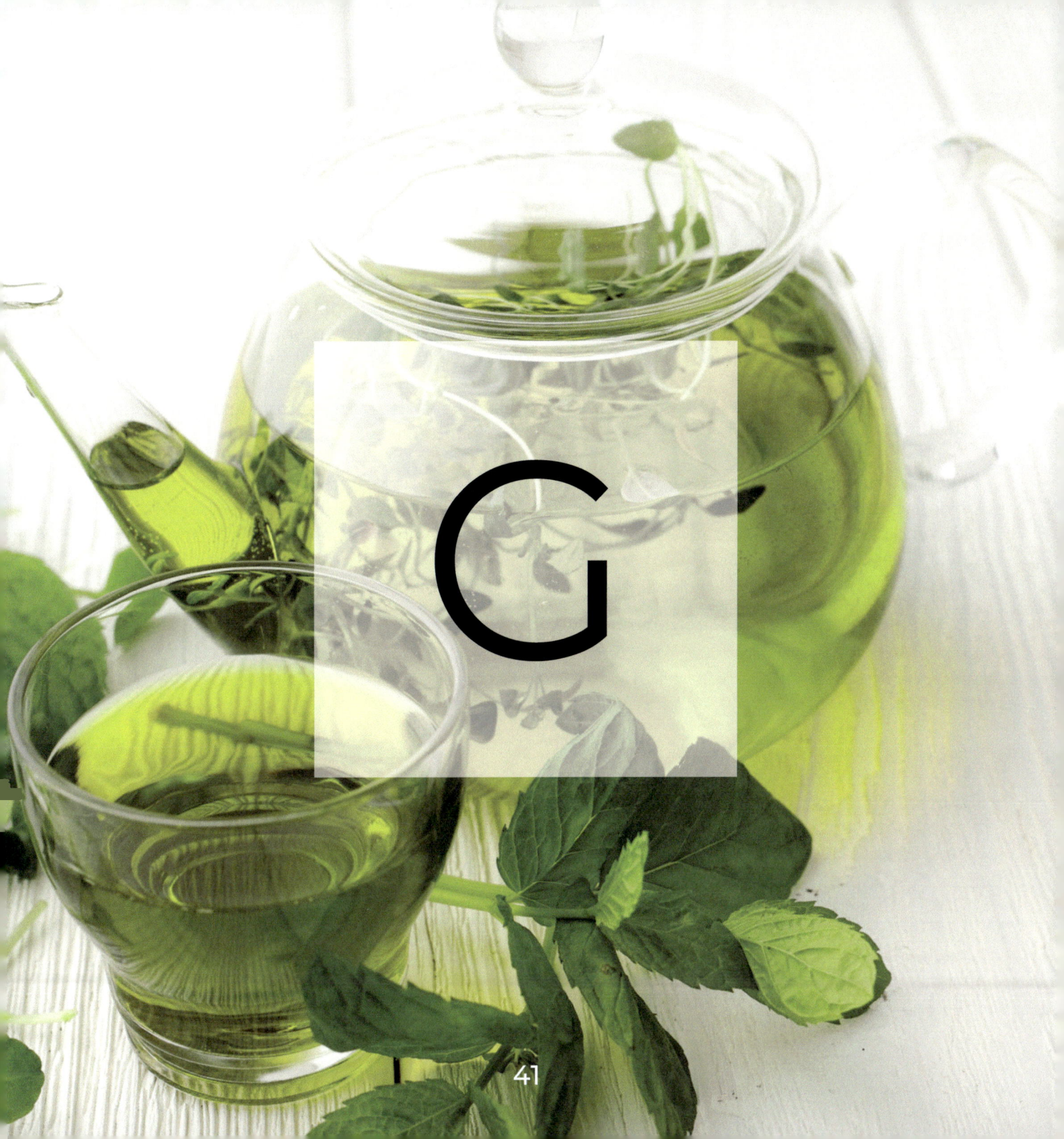

ginger

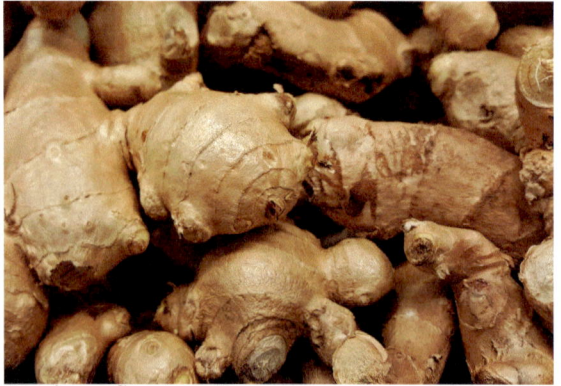

Ginger root is the rhizome (underground stem) of the flowering plant. A cousin to spices like turmeric, cardamom, and galangal, ginger is one of the most popular and healthy spices used today.

The active ingredient in ginger is gingerol, which has been used medicinally by many cultures for centuries because of its potent antioxidant and anti-inflammatory properties. Gingerol may help prevent age-related eye diseases like cataracts, glaucoma, and macular degeneration.

Eye benefits: L, O, R

In clinical studies, ginger lowered fasting blood glucose levels and hemoglobin A1C (a marker for blood sugar control), both important to decrease the risk of diabetic retinopathy. Ginger has also lowered biomarkers for oxidative stress, essential in the prevention of heart disease, stroke, and overall vascular health.

green tea

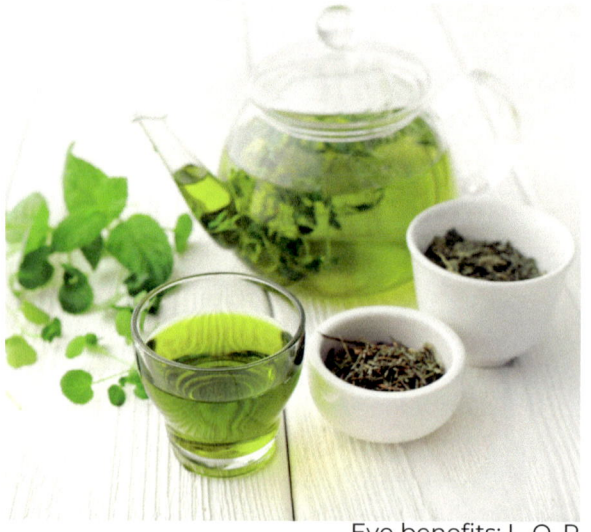

Green tea contains a host of polyphenol antioxidants that prevent cell damage and have anti-aging properties. One potent compound in green tea is a catechin called epigallocatechin-3- gallate (EGCG).

EGCG fights against oxidative damage and helps promote cellular health. In the eye, it may help protect the retina, lens, and aqueous humor, thus helping prevent age-related macular degeneration, cataract, and glaucoma.

Green tea provides a small amount of caffeine and L-theanine, which are proven important for brain health. Supporting brain health is vital for eye health, as over 50% of your brain is devoted to your visual system.

Eye benefits: L, O, R

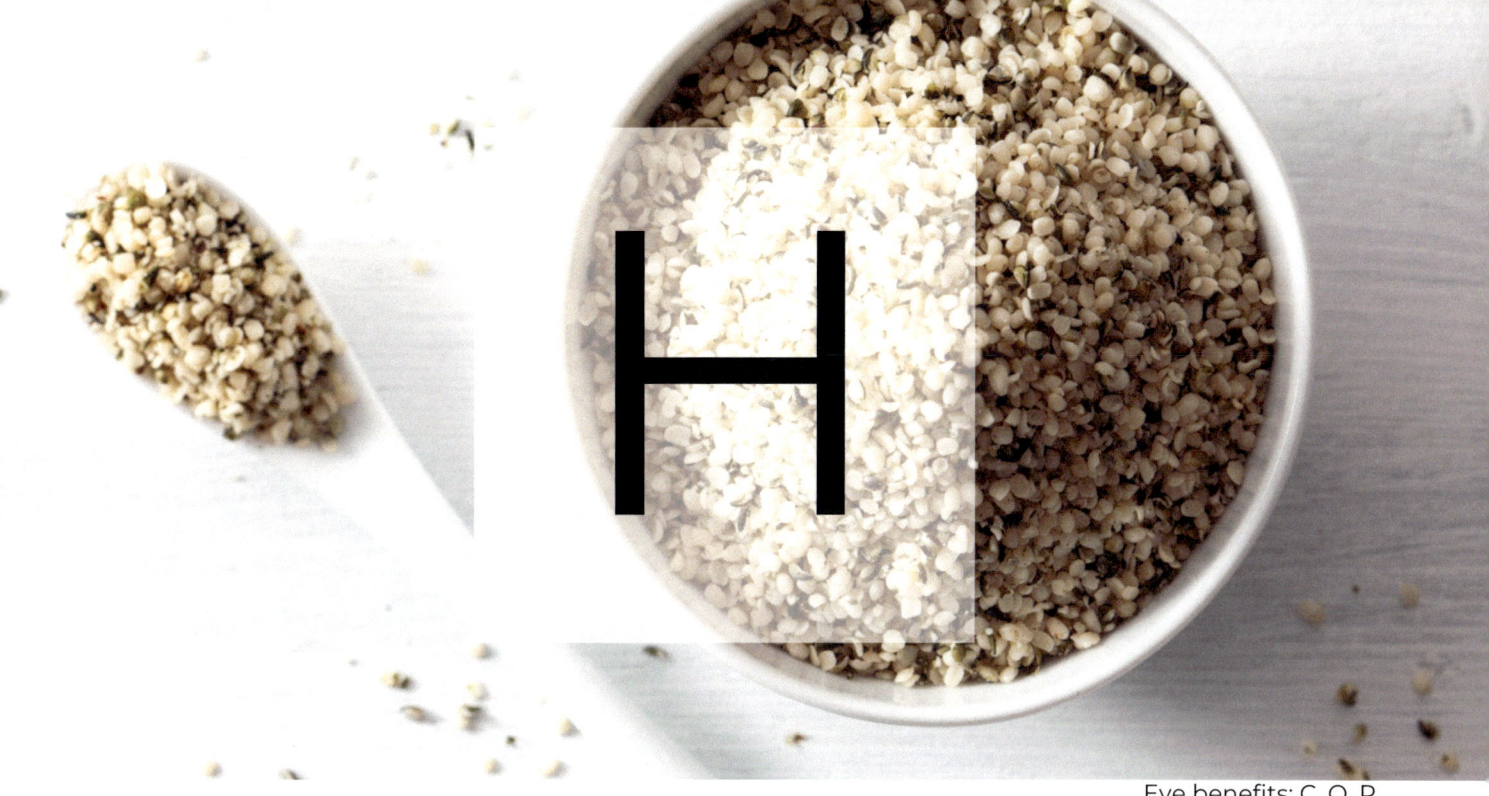

Eye benefits: C, O, R

hemp seeds

Hemp seeds come from the cannabis plant (*Cannabis sativa*). Unlike marijuana, which also comes from the cannabis plant, hemp seeds do not have significant psychoactive compounds or effects. Instead, hemp seeds, with their nutty flavor, are chock full of nutrients.

Like flax and chia, hemp seeds provide essential omega fatty acids, a combination of omega-3 (alpha-linolenic acid, ALA) and omega-6 fatty acids (gamma-linolenic acid, GLA). Together, these anti-inflammatory fatty acids help promote blood vessel, heart, and eye health.

The body can convert the ALA from hemp seeds into the essential omega-3 fatty acids, DHA and EPA, both important for retinal and ocular surface health. Omega-3s help to fight against macular degeneration and dry eye.

Hemp seeds provide several amino acids, including cysteine and glycine, two building blocks of the potent antioxidant glutathione. Hemp seeds also contain several key minerals to support metabolism and your eye health – magnesium, zinc, and iron.

I

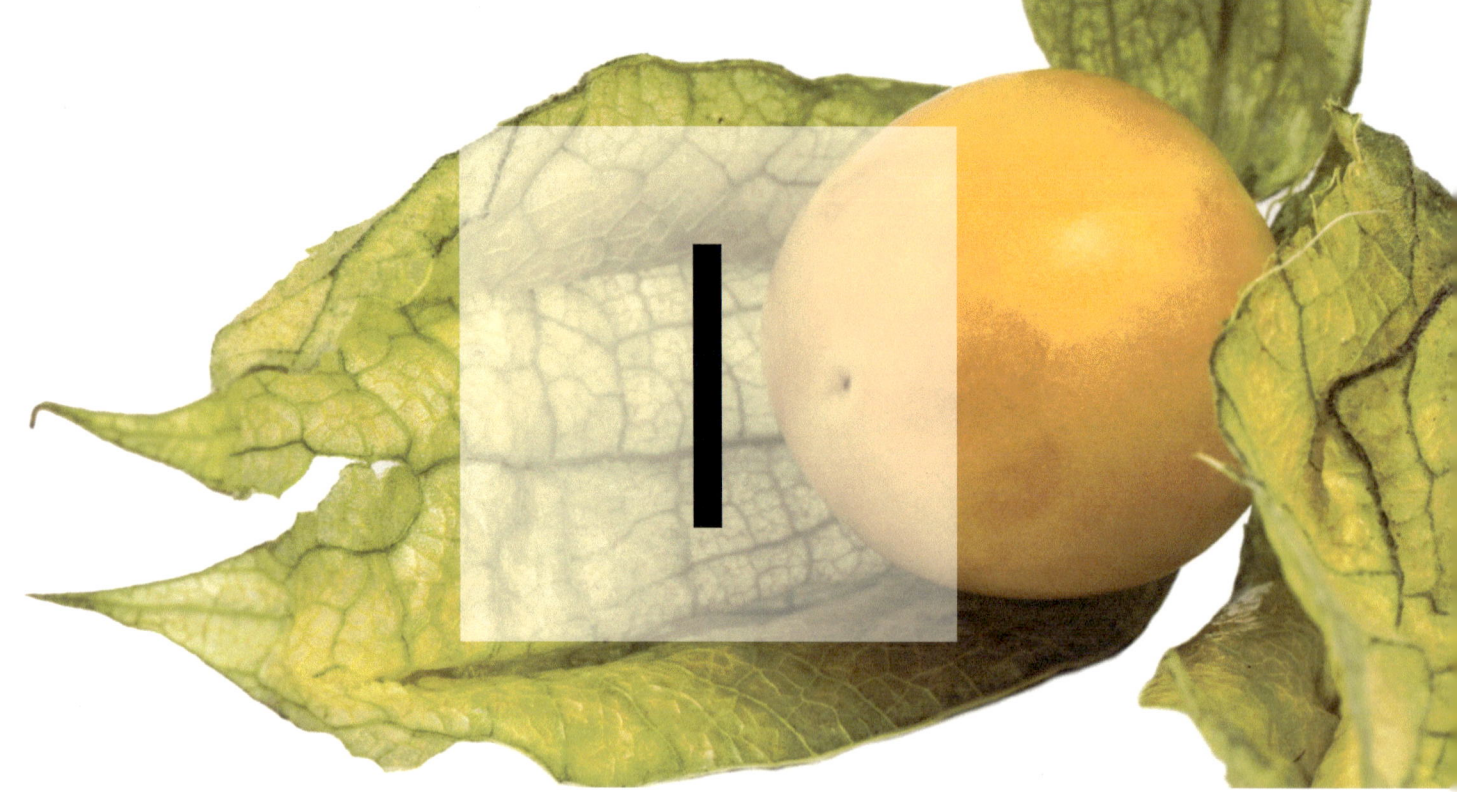

Inca berries

Eye benefits: C, L, O, R

Inca berries, also known as golden berries or cape gooseberries, differ from the more commonly known raspberries, strawberries, or blueberries. Inca berries come wrapped in a papery husk, like a tomatillo, and taste more like mango or pineapple.

Inca berries are considered a superfood, providing several nutrients excellent for your eye health. Inca berries are a rich source of vitamin A and vitamin C, potent antioxidants for the eye to protect against macular degeneration and glaucoma. Inca berries also contain lutein, a macular carotenoid that serves as an internal UV and blue-blocking filter, as well as beta carotene that can be converted to Vitamin A to fight against night blindness and retinal disease.

Inca berries provide several B vitamins - namely thiamine (B1), riboflavin (B2), and niacin B3) - essential for energy production by your mitochondria and brain health. Finally, these tropical berries are an excellent source of fiber, with 6 grams per 1 cup serving, which is important to support gut health and digestion. They are best eaten fully ripe, without any green spots.

J

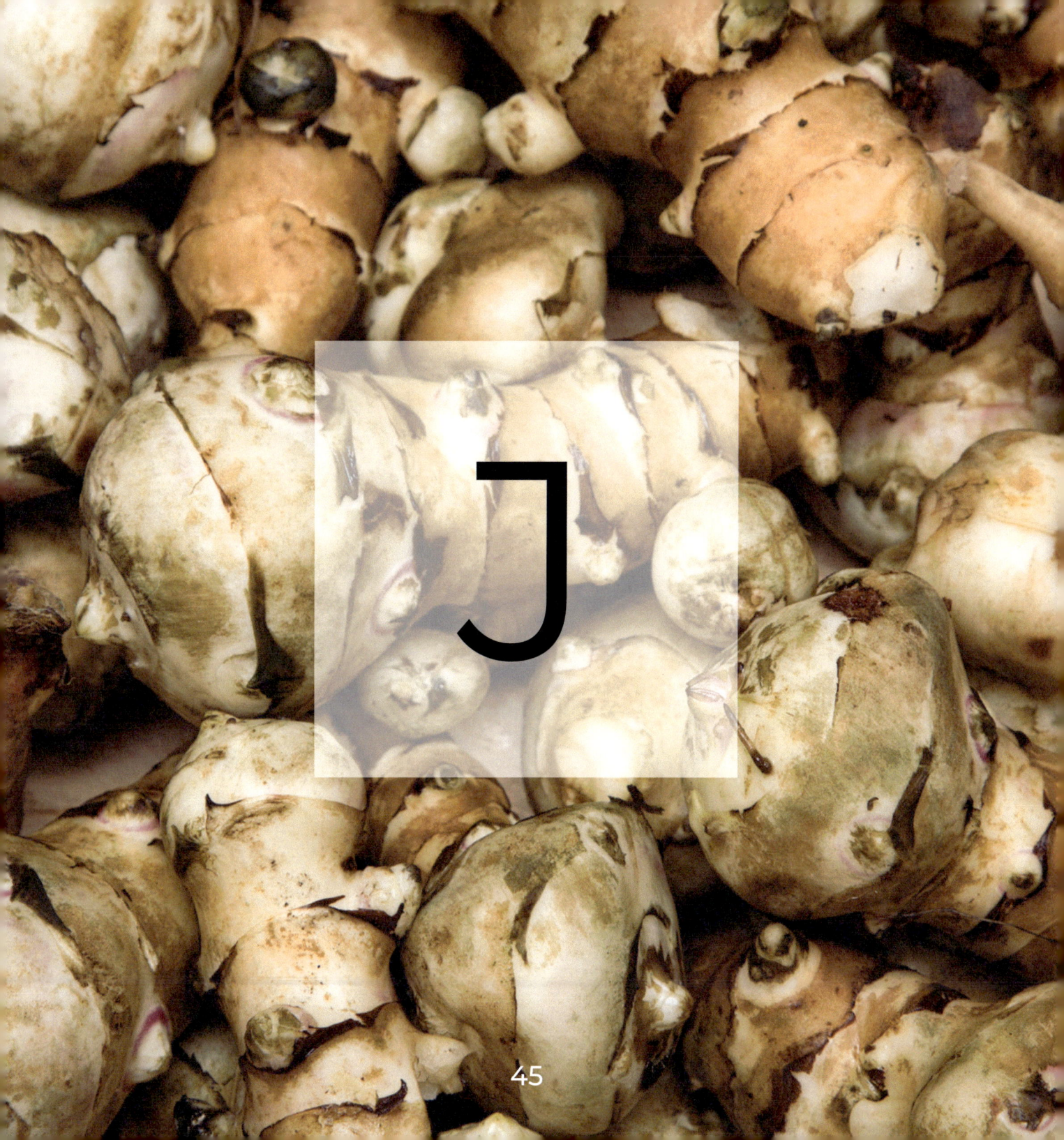

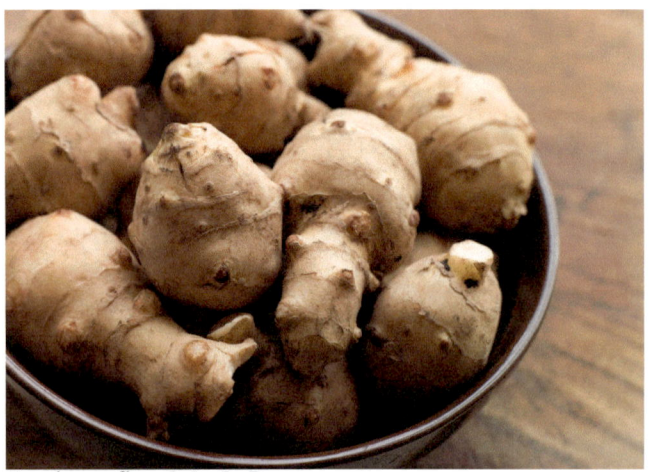

Jerusalem artichoke

Jerusalem artichoke has several important eye health benefits. Firstly, it provides vitamin C that acts as an antioxidant to limit the damage caused by free radicals. Antioxidants may aid in the prevention of age-related cataracts and macular degeneration. Vitamin C is also essential for the synthesis of collagen, the building block of the eye.

Jerusalem artichoke also provides two B vitamins, thiamine (B1) and niacin (B3), which are important for mitochondrial energy production.

Eye benefits: C, L, O, R

Finally, Jerusalem artichoke is excellent for gut health because it contains fiber for optimal digestion and provides inulin which acts as a prebiotic to feed and support your gut microbiome.

jicama

Jicama is a root vegetable with papery, golden-brown skin and a crunchy white interior. It has a slightly nutty and sweet flavor. Jicama provides the eye with a high concentration of vitamin C. Vitamin C is essential for the eye's collagen structure and acts as an antioxidant to protect against many age-related eye diseases like glaucoma, cataract, and macular degeneration.

Jicama provides folate, magnesium, and potassium, with smaller amounts of vitamin E, thiamine (B1), riboflavin (B2), pyridoxine (B6), zinc, and copper, all critical nutrients for optimal energy production and metabolism. For gut health, jicama is excellent in its high fiber and water content. It also has inulin, a prebiotic that supports a healthy gut microbiome.

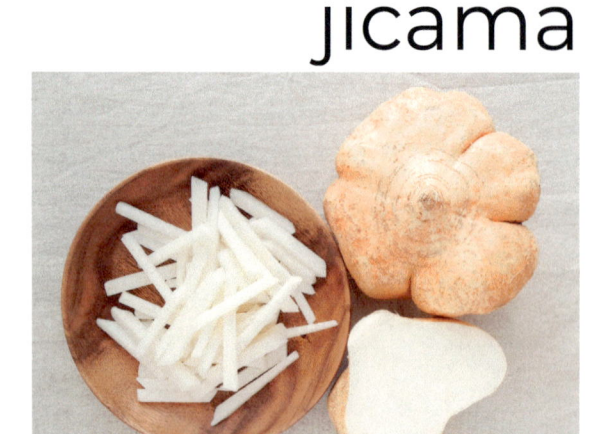

Eye benefits: C, L, O, R

K

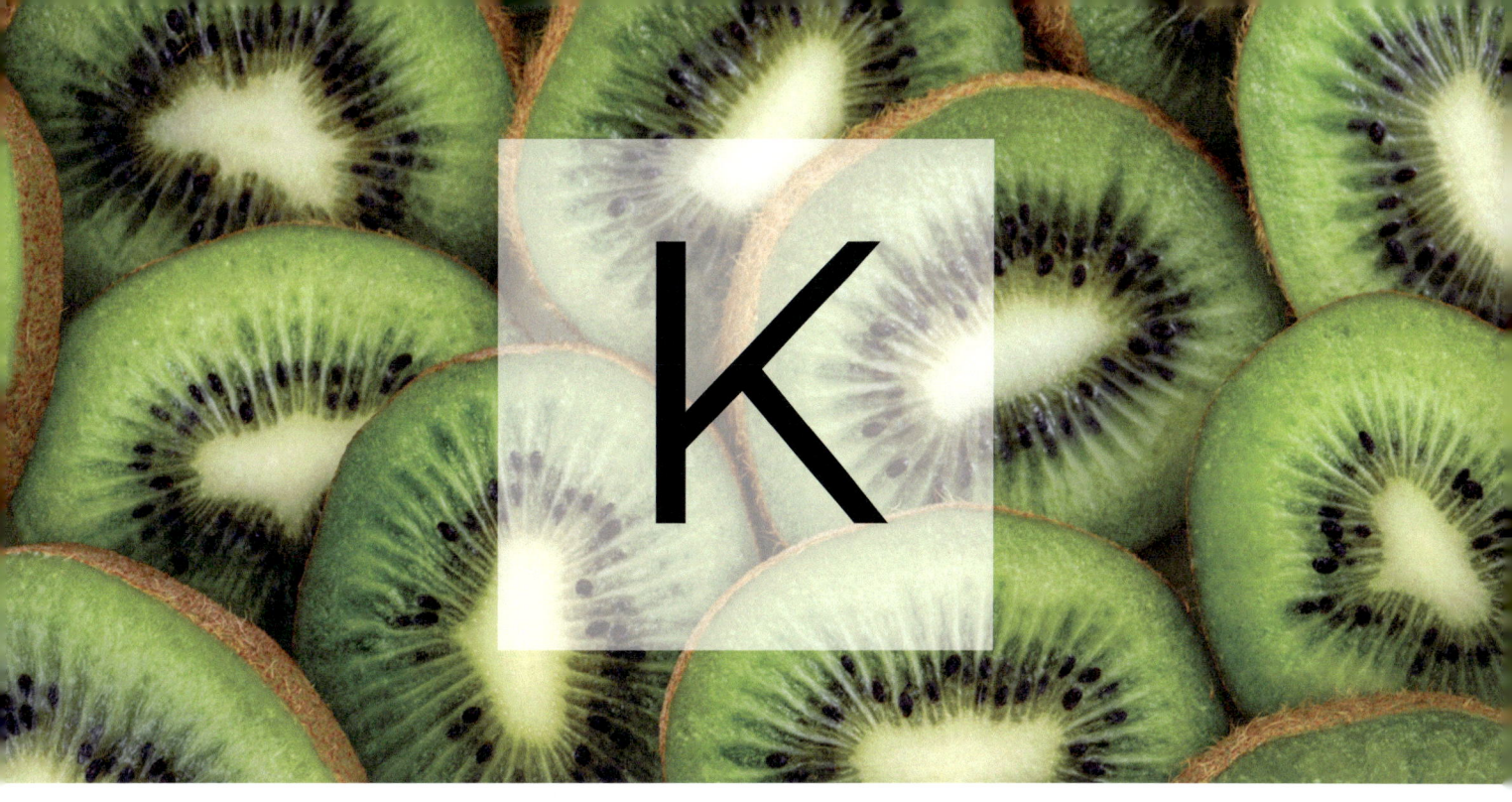

kiwi

Eye benefits: C, L, R

Kiwi is named after the kiwi bird found in New Zealand because of its fuzzy brown skin. This oval fruit has a soft green pulp speckled with seeds and has a tangy, sweet taste.

Kiwi contains many nutrients key to healthy vision. Kiwi provides lutein, zeaxanthin, and beta carotene, carotenoids that help protect against macular degeneration, a leading cause of vision loss. One study showed that people who ate 3 compared to 1.5 fruits daily had a decreased risk of macular degeneration.

Kiwi is an excellent source of vitamin C, with one cup providing 273% of your daily requirement. Vitamin C is an antioxidant to protect against age-related eye diseases; it also helps boost your immune system and supports the production of collagen, the eye's structural building block.

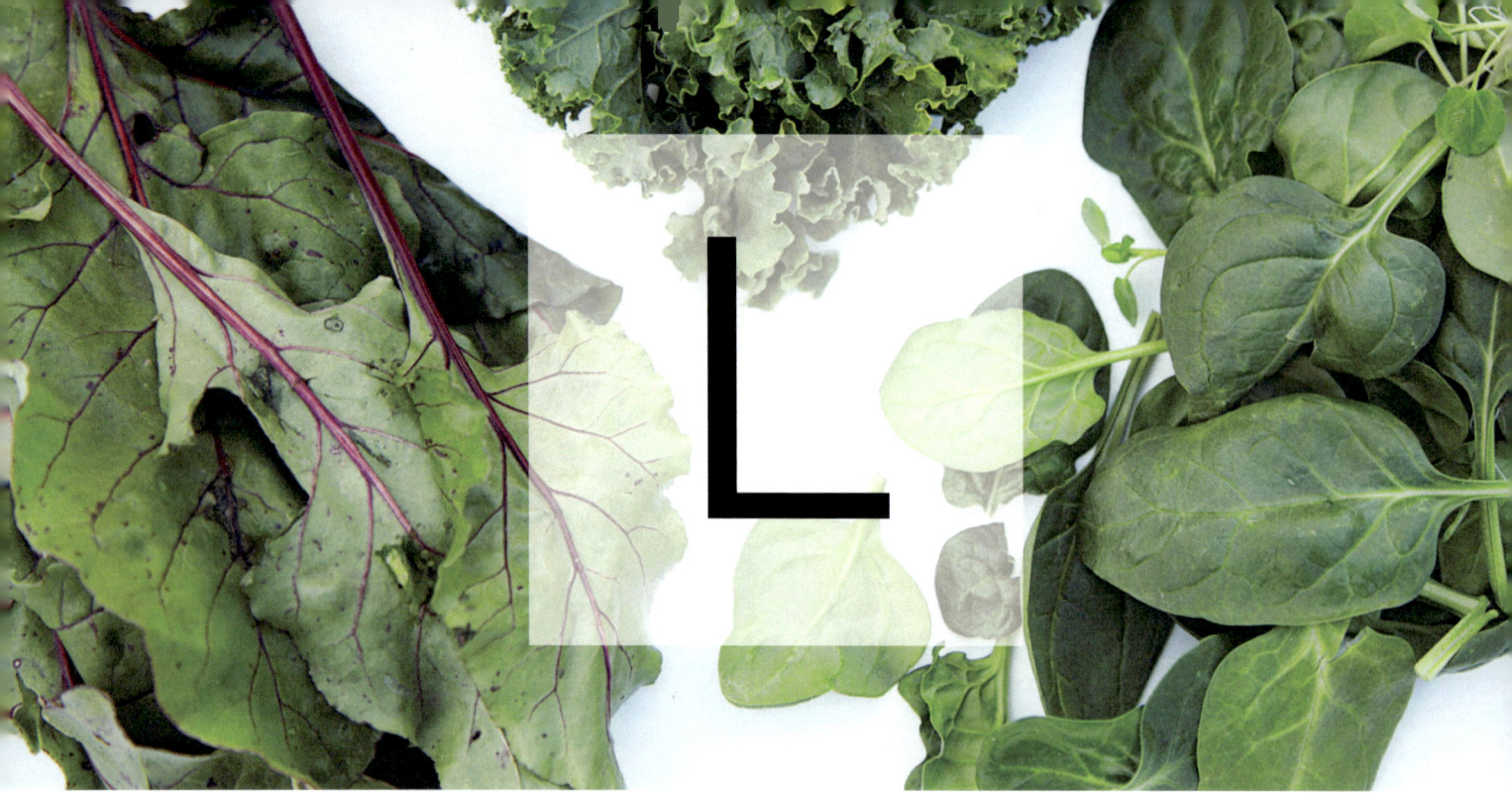

leafy greens

Eye benefits: C, L, O, R

Dark green, leafy vegetables are superfoods for eye health. These vegetables provide high concentrations of lutein and zeaxanthin. Studies have shown that people who consume high amounts of these macular carotenoids are protected against vision loss from macular degeneration, a leading cause of blindness. Not only do these macular carotenoids provide antioxidant protection, but they are also anti-inflammatory.

In addition, green leafy vegetables are an excellent source of vitamin A. Vitamin A is needed for processing light energy by retinal photoreceptors. Vitamin A deficiency, a severe condition known as xerophthalmia, can result in night blindness. Vitamin A is also important for the ocular surface's health; its deficiency can lead to severe dry eye and even corneal ulceration. Finally, Vitamin A can help protect the eye's delicate structures from UV light and oxidative damage.

Many other nutrients can be found in leafy greens that benefit your eyes, including vitamins C, K, and E, folate (B9), and potassium, to name a few. Leafy greens are also an excellent source of fiber, helpful for digestion and gut health.

The leafy greens best for eye health include:

-Kale

-Spinach

-Romaine lettuce

-Swiss chard

-Collard greens

-Dandelion greens

-Mustard greens

-Turnip greens

-Arugula

-Watercress

-Bok choy

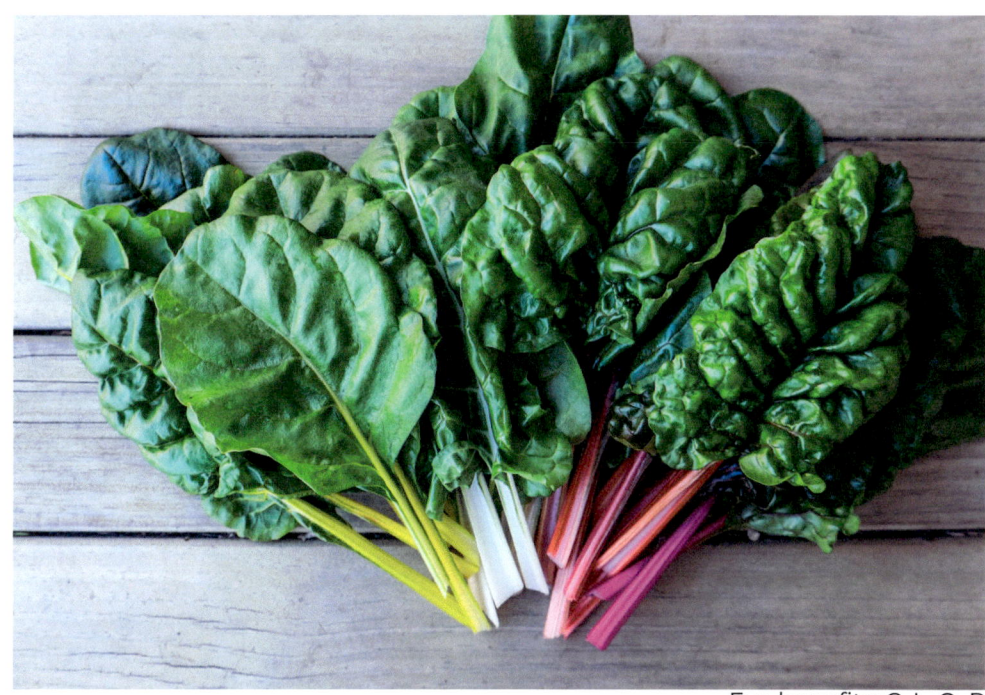

Eye benefits: C, L, O, R

Some of these leafy greens are also part of the Brassica family and provide glucosinolates, sulfur-based compounds that are anti-inflammatory and important in the detoxification pathways.

Not only do many of these leafy greens support eye health, but they are also beneficial for brain health. Remember that at least 50% of the brain is dedicated to our visual systems, so supporting a healthy brain also protects your vision!

M

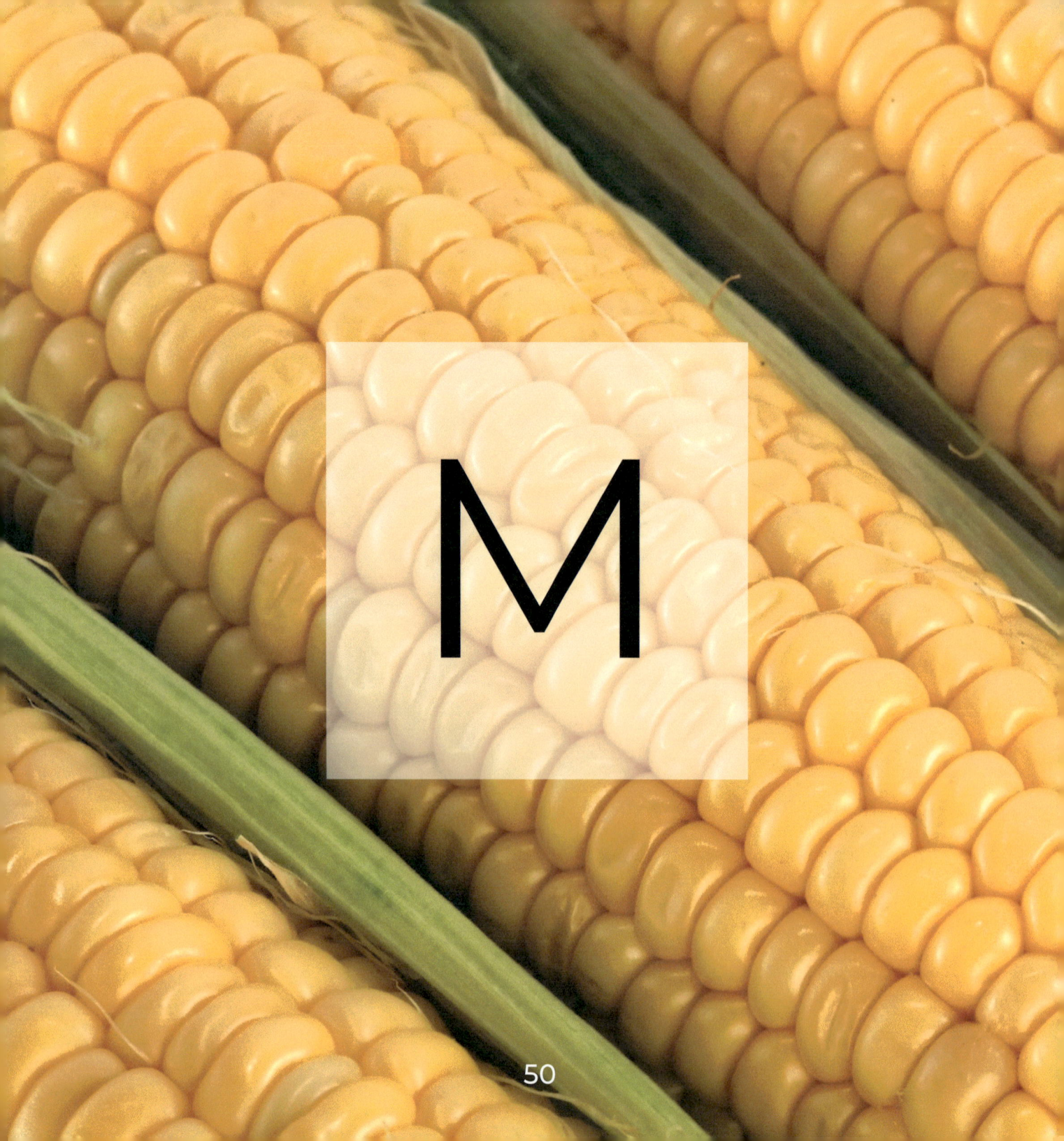

maize

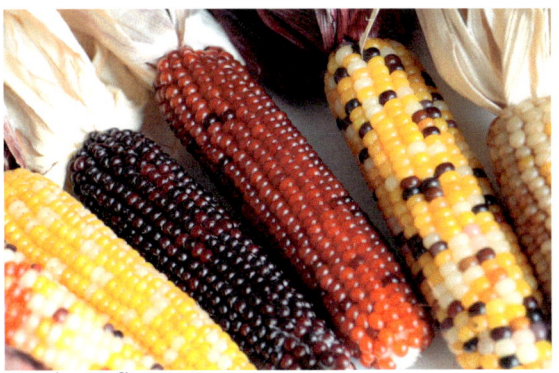

Maize, or corn, is typically yellow but can also be found in white, red, orange, blue, purple, and black. Yellow maize contains one of the highest concentrations of the macular carotenoids, lutein and zeaxanthin, of any food. The word zeaxanthin is derived from the corn plant, Zea mays. These yellow pigments are deposited into the center of the retina, the macula, to protect it from oxidative damage from free radicals and light toxicity. Both lutein and zeaxanthin are critical in the prevention of macular degeneration.

Eye benefits: L, R

The colorful shades of maize, particularly the blue, purple, and black varieties, have additional pigmented nutrients called anthocyanins. Anthocyanins help protect against oxidative stress and have been found to be beneficial for macular degeneration.

mushrooms

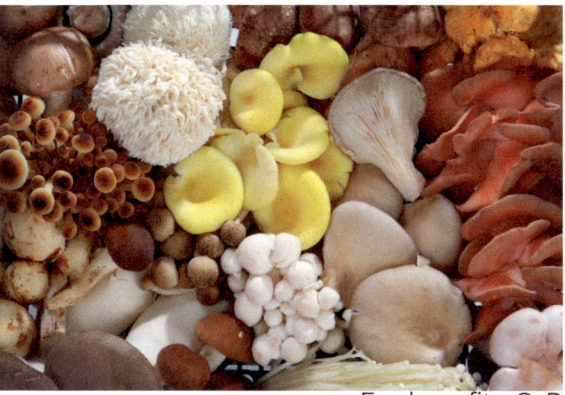

Mushrooms are fungi that come in unique sizes, shapes, colors, and tastes. Mushrooms have rich nutritional profiles. Mushrooms provide riboflavin (B2), niacin (B3), and pantothenic acid (B5) – all critical for optimal energy production. Mushrooms are also a good source of minerals - selenium, copper, and potassium - all important for eye health.

Some mushrooms provide vitamin D, which plays a vital role in the immune system and is anti-inflammatory. Low vitamin D levels have been associated with macular degeneration.

Eye benefits: O, R

Many mushroom varieties are brain and eye-healthy, such as reishi, lion's mane (yamabushitake), maitake, shiitake, and tiger milk. Reishi mushroom spores were demonstrated to protect against cell death in the retina by inhibiting certain genes.

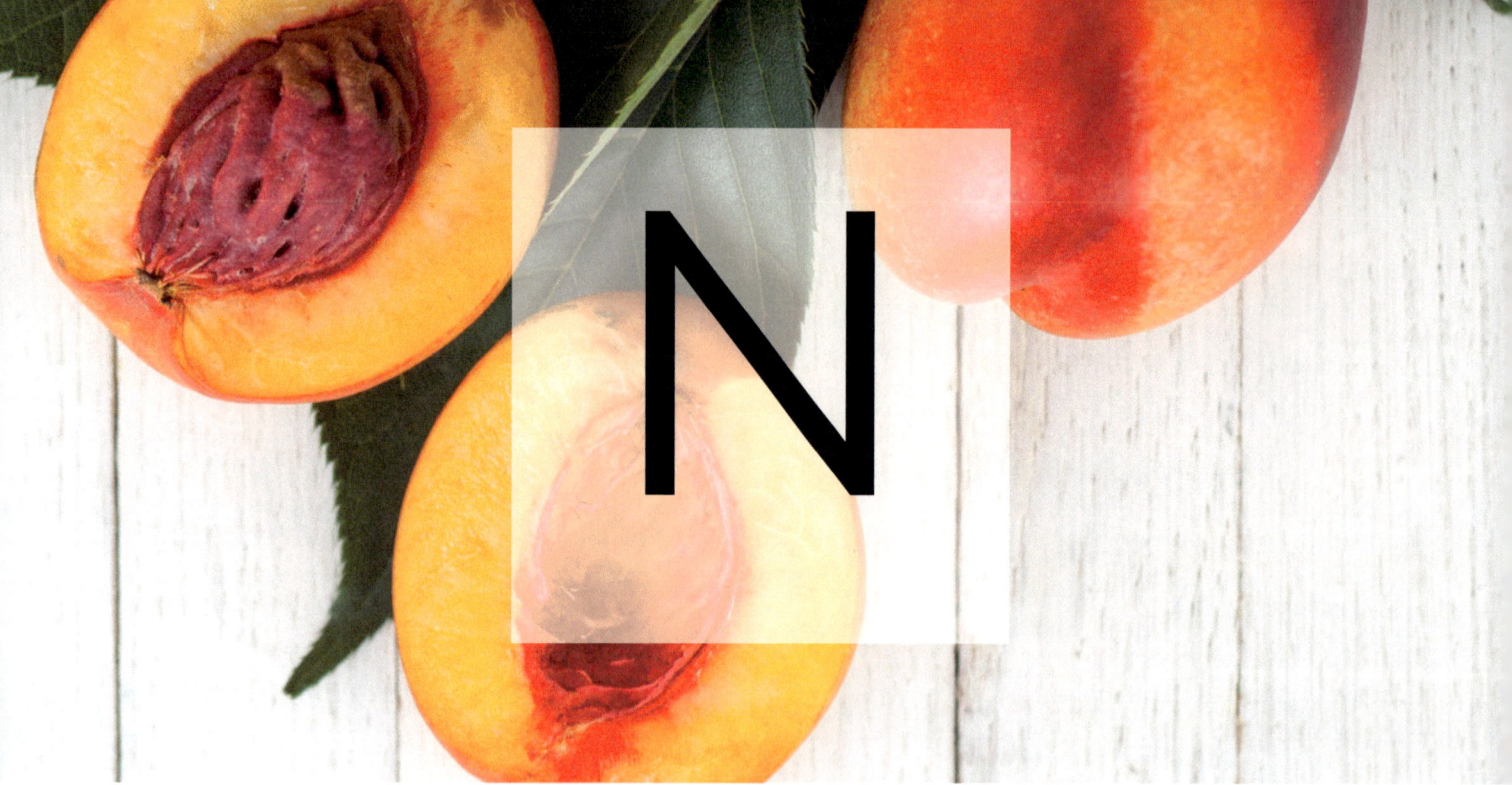

Eye benefits: C, L, O, R

nectarine

Nectarine is a stone fruit with smooth skin and juicy, orange pulp. Nectarine is an excellent source of vitamin C, an antioxidant to fight against cataracts and macular degeneration, and an essential nutrient for healthy collagen in the eye. Nectarine provides niacin (B3), necessary for energy production in the eye. Nectarine also contains several vital minerals for eye health: copper, potassium, zinc, iron, magnesium, manganese, and phosphorus.

Nectarine, with its bright orange color, is a wonderful source of carotenoids- vitamin A, lutein, and zeaxanthin, all beneficial for healthy vision. Vitamin A deficiency can result in night blindness, decreased vision, and dry eyes. Lutein and zeaxanthin help prevent cataracts and macular degeneration. Finally, nectarine is also a good source of prebiotic fiber, promoting healthy digestion and the gut microbiome.

Nectarine is a cousin to the fuzzy-skinned peach, also a stone fruit. Peach has a similar nutritional profile to nectarine and is also excellent for promoting eye health.

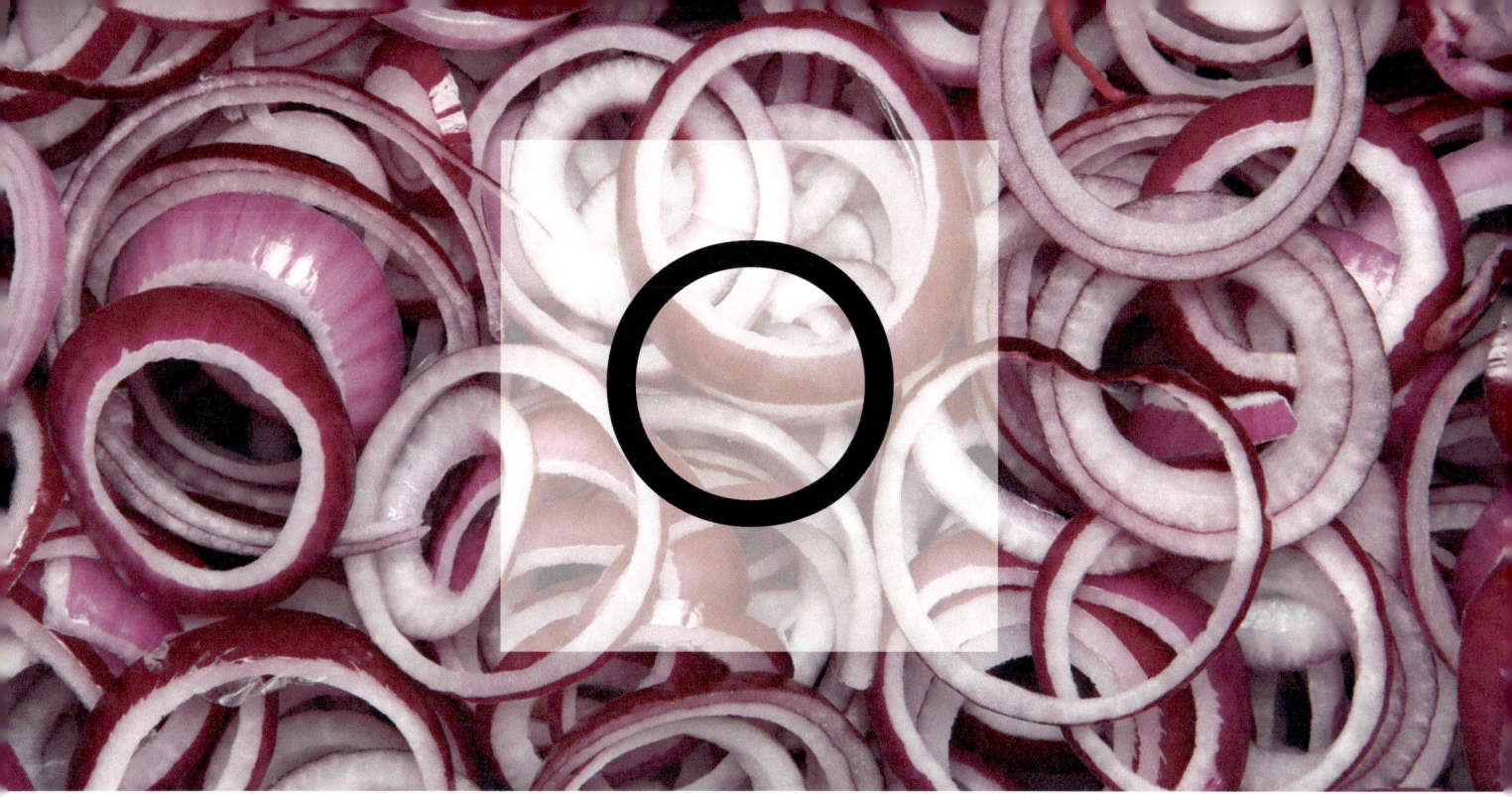

onion

Eye benefits: C, L, O, R

Onion is a member of the Allium family of flowering plants and a cousin to garlic, leeks, chives, and shallots. Onion is high in several vitamins, minerals, and polyphenols crucial for eye health.

Firstly, onion is rich in vitamin C, essential for the eye's collagen production, tissue repair, and immune health. Vitamin C is also a key antioxidant for the eye to protect against damage caused by free radicals.

Onion is a good source of B vitamins such as folate (B9) and pyridoxine (B6) which are essential for nerve function, red blood cell production, and energy metabolism.

Onion contains high amounts of quercetin, a polyphenol that is a strong immune modulator and reduces inflammation. Red onion has an even higher concentration of quercetin.

Quercetin can also be found in other vegetables and fruits such as apple, berries, caper, plum, red wine, kale, asparagus, and broccoli.

P

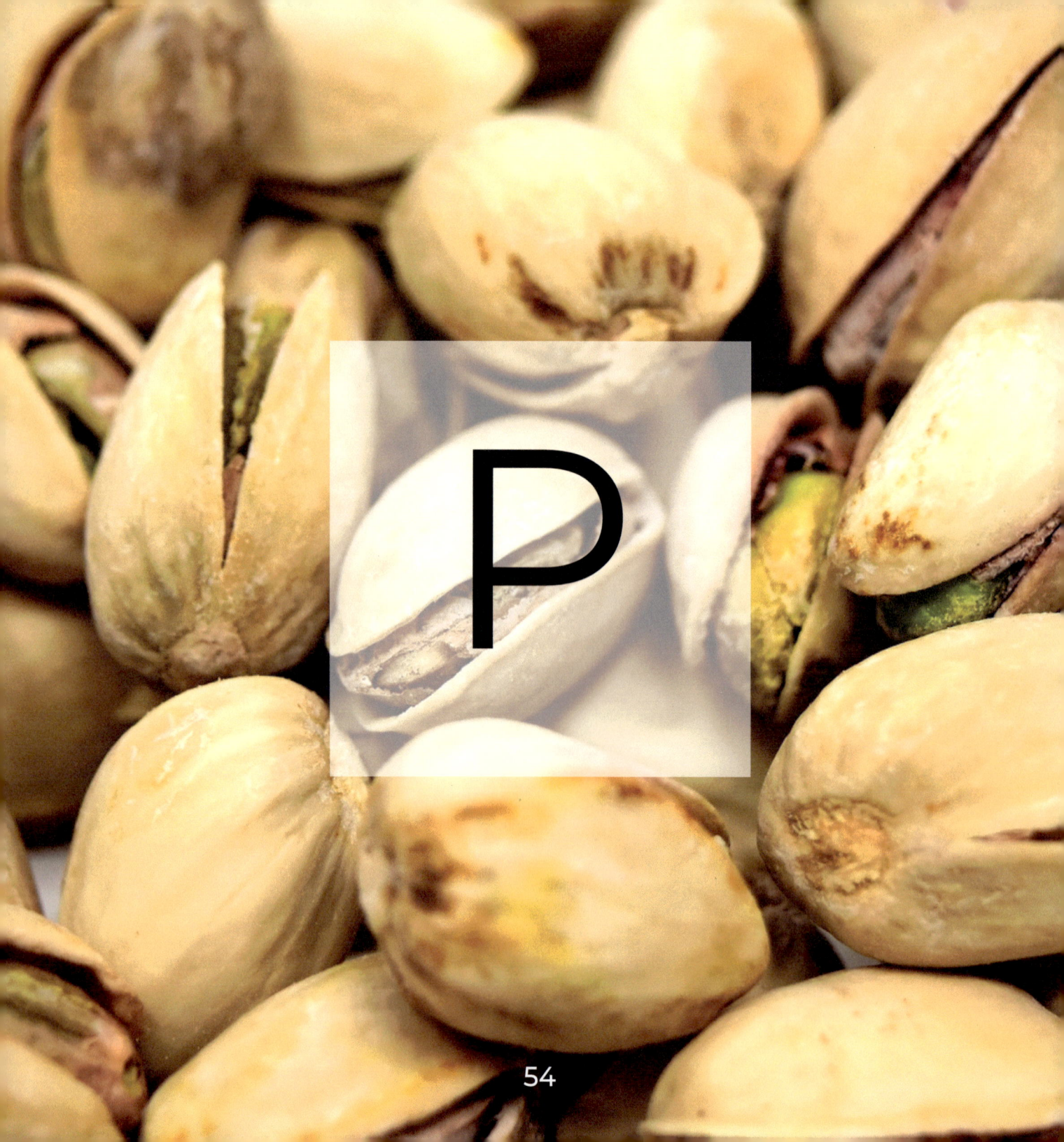

paprika

Eye benefits: C, L, R

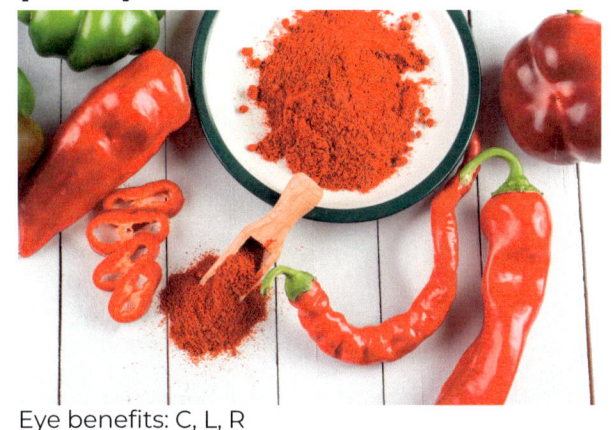

Paprika is a colorful spice made from dried peppers from the Capsicum family, such as bell, chili, poblano, cayenne, or Aleppo peppers. Paprika can be red, orange, or yellow in color and comes in sweet, hot, or smoked varieties. Paprika is very high in carotenoids, especially lutein and zeaxanthin, that protect the retina and lens against oxidative stress from UV or blue light and other forms of oxidative stress. Paprika is an excellent source of beta carotene, a precursor to vitamin A and essential for corneal, conjunctival, and retinal health.

Another carotenoid in paprika is capsanthin, shown to raise levels of good cholesterol, HDL; HDL is important in transporting lutein and zeaxanthin. The spice also provides vitamin E, an antioxidant useful in the fight against cataracts and macular degeneration.

parsley

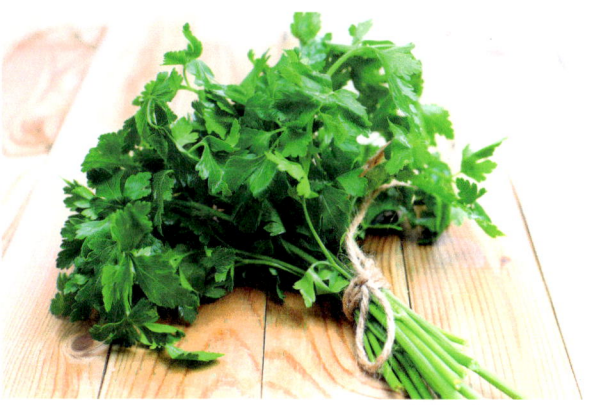

Parsley is a fragrant, bright green culinary herb with a slightly bitter taste. Parsley provides key carotenoids, including lutein, zeaxanthin, and beta-carotene.

Parsley provides a high concentration of Vitamins C and K, the former being an important antioxidant for the eyes and the latter for healthy blood clotting and prevention of excessive bleeding.

Parsley is particularly rich in a class of antioxidants known as flavonoids. The two main flavonoids in parsley include myricetin and apigenin. Apigenin has been shown to stabilize blood vessels and may play a key role in preventing conditions such as diabetic retinopathy and macular degeneration.

Eye benefits: C, L, R

pistachio

Most nuts support eye health, though pistachios stand out as one of the most nutrient-dense. Pistachios provide high concentrations of the macular carotenoids, lutein and zeaxanthin. These yellow-pigmented nutrients protect your eyes against damage from ultraviolet and blue light.

Pistachios provide polyphenols and tocopherols (vitamin E) that act as powerful antioxidants to protect your vision from age-related conditions like cataracts, glaucoma, and macular degeneration.

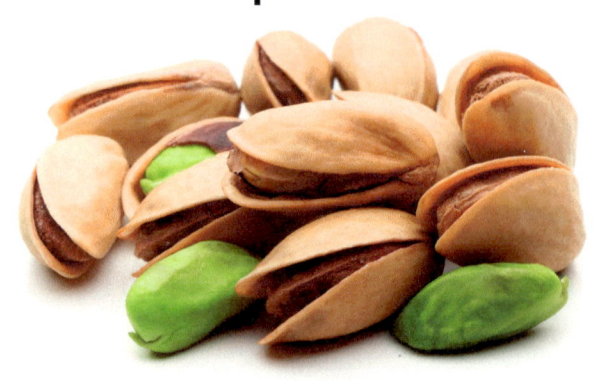

Eye benefits: C, L, O, R

Pistachios are also a rich source of protein. Pistachio nuts also provide several essential and non-essential amino acids, like L-arginine. The body converts L-arginine into nitric oxide, a molecule that dilates blood vessels and promotes blood flow to the eye and brain.

pomegranate

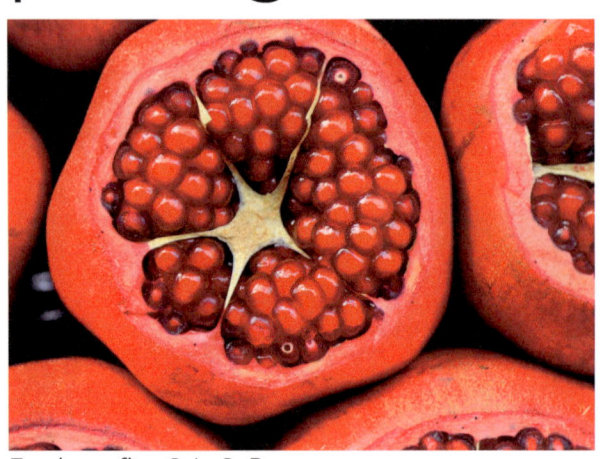

Pomegranate is one of the healthiest and tastiest of fruits. It has hundreds of red, edible seeds called arils that burst with a sweet flavor.

Pomegranate provides polyphenol antioxidants that have anti-aging and anti-inflammatory properties. Pomegranate has two unique substances: punicalagin and punicic acid; these are powerful antioxidants with three times the potency of green tea and red wine. In addition, pomegranate provides several essential eye nutrients, namely vitamins C and K, folate (B9), and potassium.

Eye benefits: C, L, O, R

One caveat about pomegranate – the arils and juice have a high sugar content (glycemic index), so they are best consumed in small quantities so as not to raise blood sugar.

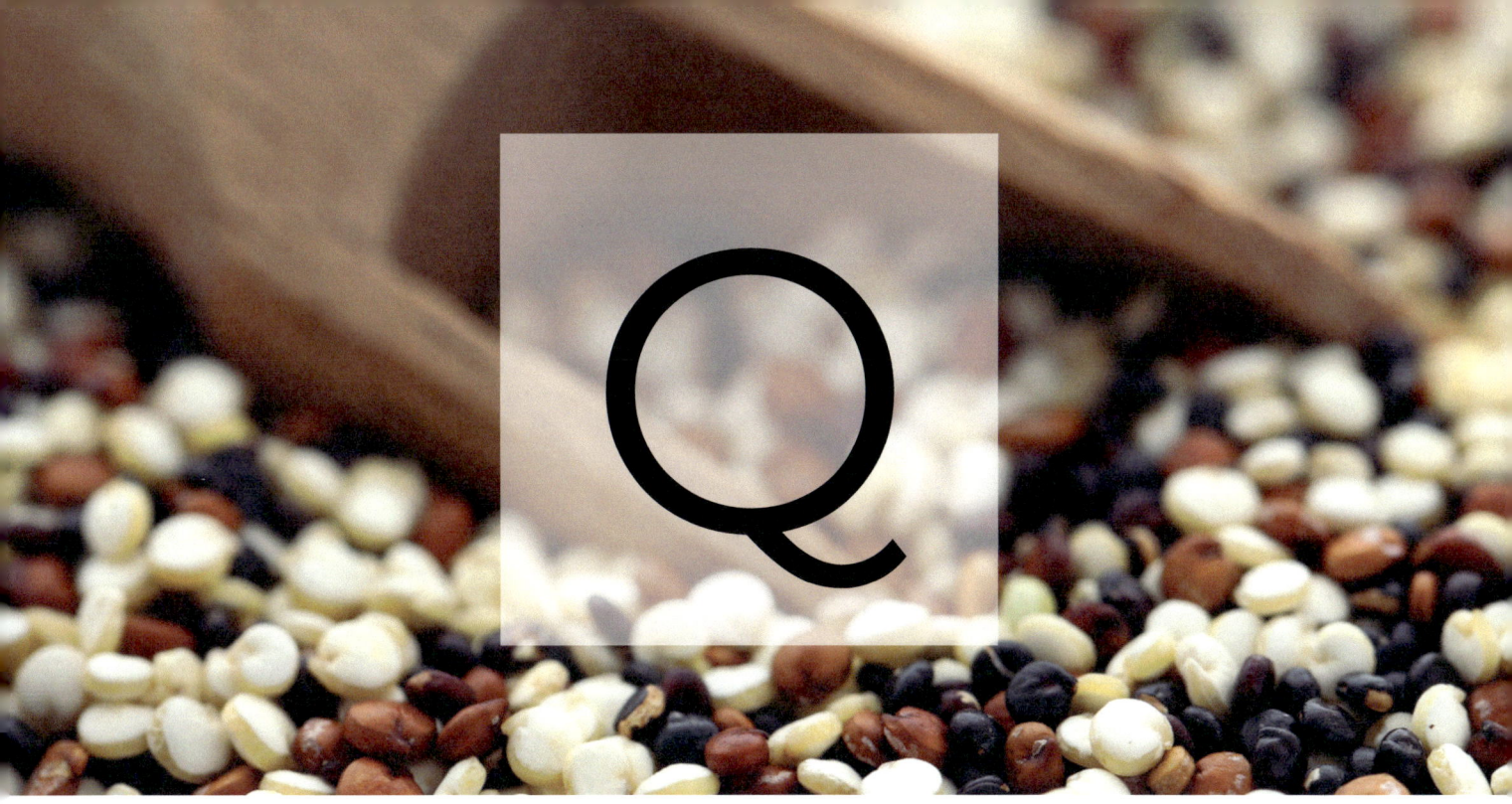

quinoa

Eye benefits: O, R

Quinoa is an edible seed native to the Andes mountains. Quinoa comes in white, red, or black varieties and can often substitute for grains in many dishes. Quinoa is a "superfood" because it provides many nutrients and health benefits.

Quinoa contains high amounts of quercetin and kaempferol, two polyphenol flavonoids that are potent antioxidants and anti-inflammatory. Quinoa is an excellent source of several B vitamins essential for converting food into energy and nerve health – thiamine (B1), riboflavin (B2), and folic acid (B9).

Quinoa provides the critical mineral magnesium, important for over 600 enzymatic reactions in the body, including energy metabolism in the eye. Quinoa also contains several other minerals for eye health- zinc, iron, phosphorus, potassium, and manganese.

In addition, quinoa is an excellent plant-based source of protein and all nine essential amino acids. Finally, quinoa is a good source of insoluble fiber that aids digestion and gut health.

R

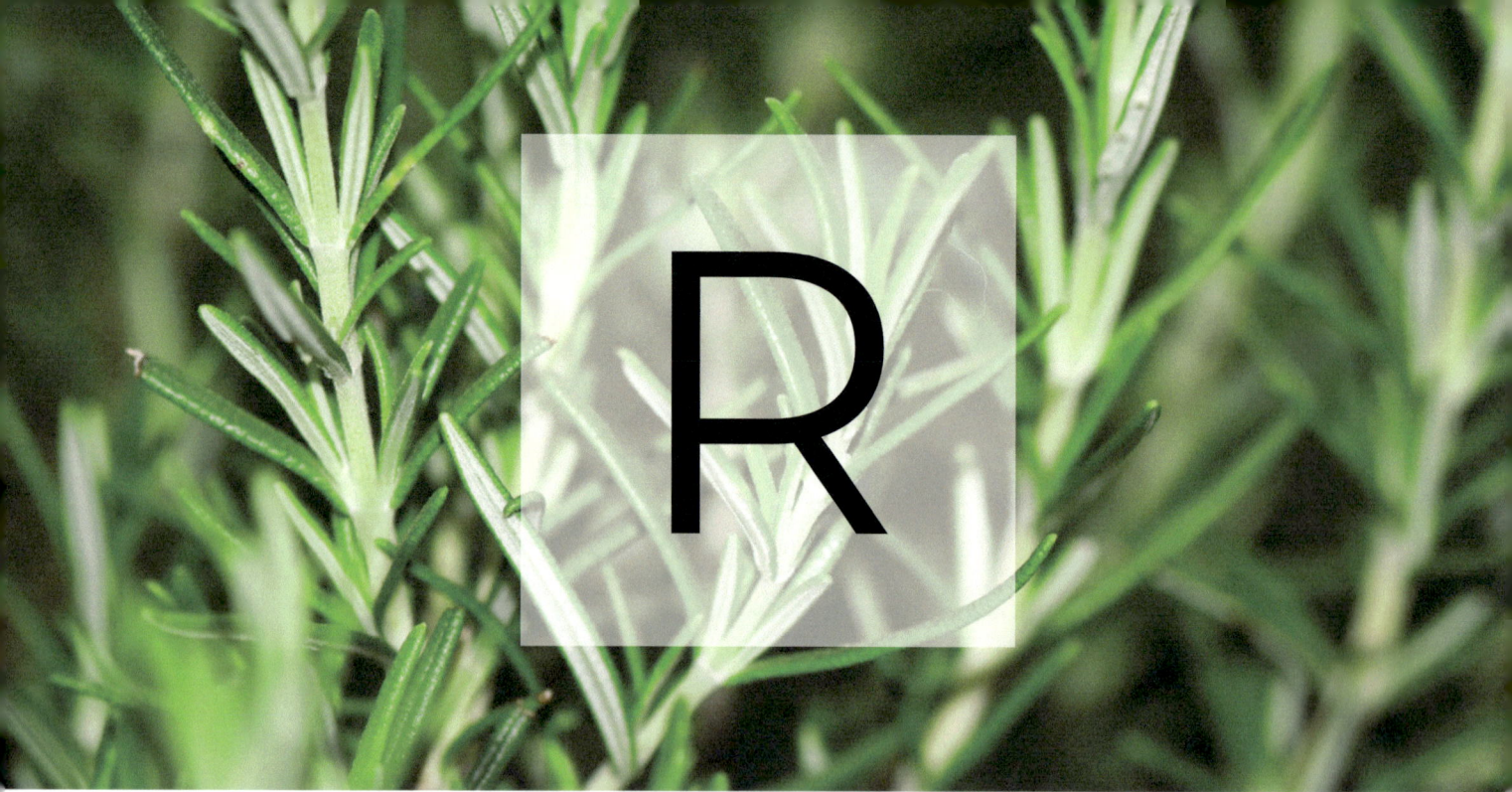

rosemary

Eye benefits: R

Rosemary is an herb that has long been used for its culinary, aromatic, and medicinal properties. Rosemary adds fragrance and flavor to foods and can also be used as tea or oil.

Rosemary's active ingredient is carnosic acid, an antioxidant shown to protect the retina from light toxicity and degeneration in cell culture and animal studies. It has been proposed that rosemary may protect retinal photoreceptors from oxidative damage from macular degeneration and retinitis pigmentosa.

In addition to carnosic acid, rosemary also contains rosmarinic acid, an antioxidant and anti-inflammatory compound that helps boost the immune system.

Beyond eye health, rosemary has been touted to be beneficial for brain health. Its aroma has been shown to boost a person's concentration, memory, performance, and speed. Rosemary has been used in the prevention and treatment of neurodegenerative diseases.

S

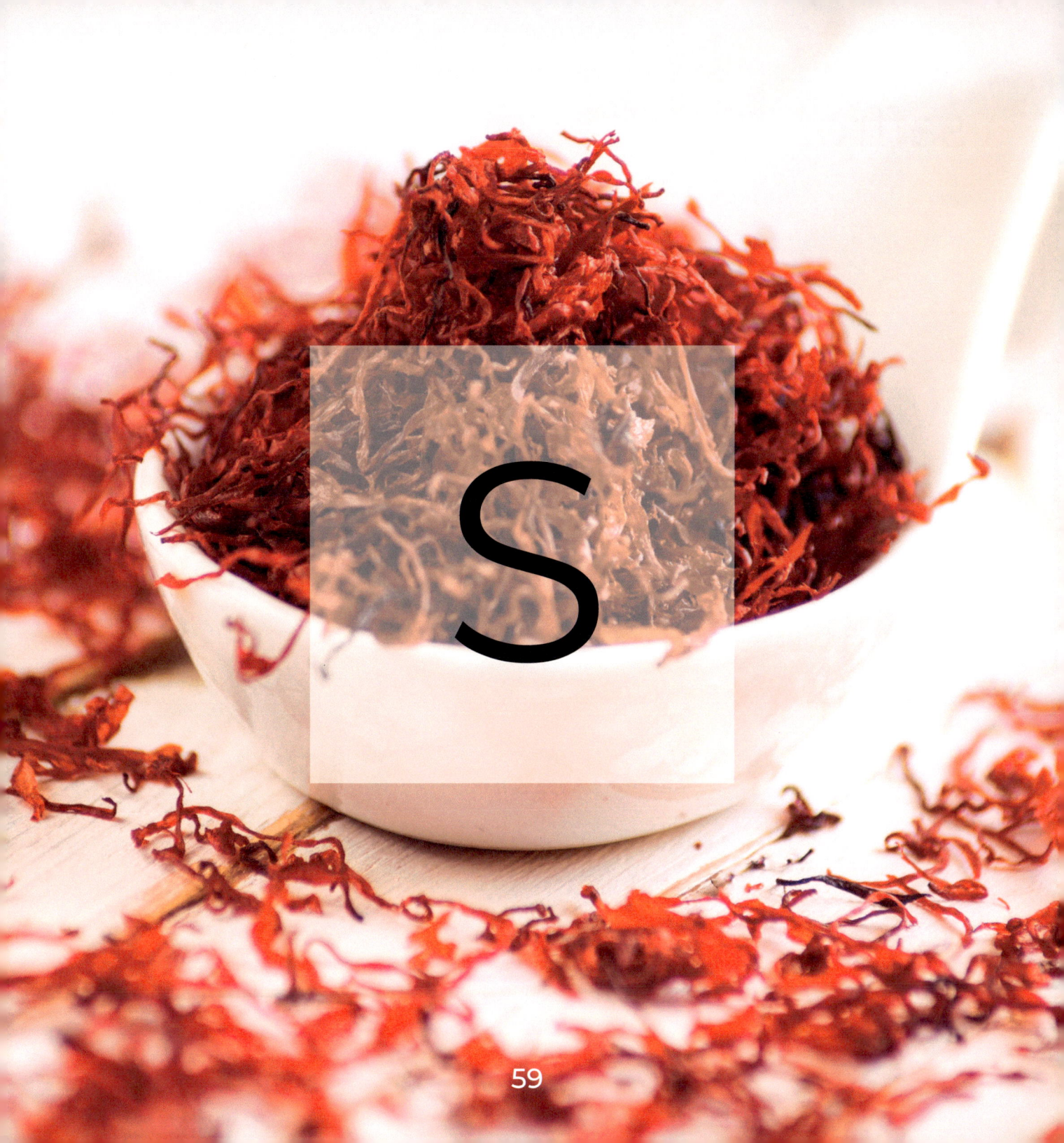

saffron

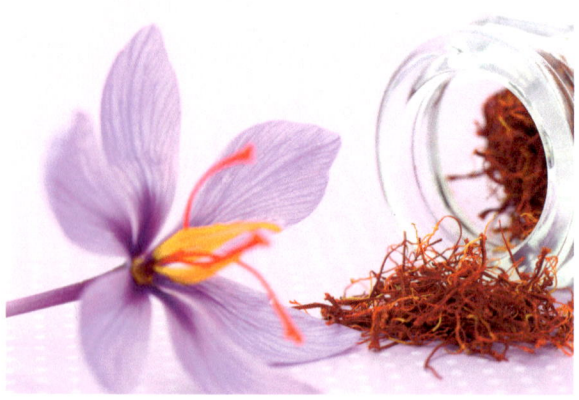

Eye benefits: R

Saffron is a bright orange-red spice from the stigma of the *Crocus sativus* flower. With its high concentration of polyphenol and carotenoid antioxidants, saffron offers many health benefits. Saffron's active compounds include crocin, crocetin, safranal, and kaempferol.

Saffron protects against free radical damage linked to age-related macular degeneration (AMD). At a dose of 20 mg taken daily for one year, saffron has been shown to improve visual acuity and visual function in adults with AMD.

Saffron also helps regulate blood sugar levels and improves insulin sensitivity, thus decreasing the risk for diabetic retinopathy.

seaweed

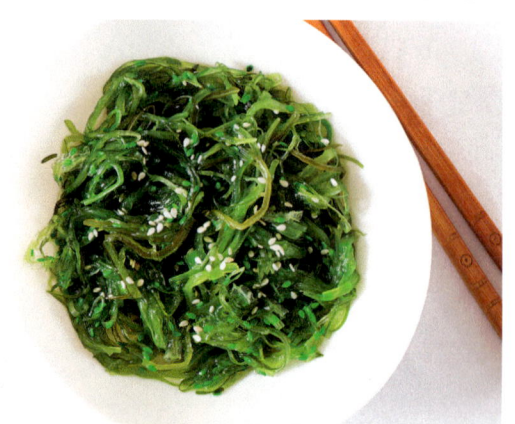

Seaweed and sea vegetables are algae that come in a variety of colors, shapes, and sizes. Seaweed is an excellent source of key minerals essential for enzymatic function and energy production- iodine, copper, iron, manganese, zinc, and magnesium.

Seaweed provides vitamins A, C, and E, three key antioxidants to protect your eye from cell damage. A type of brown seaweed called wakame contains a carotenoid called fucoxanthin that is over 13.5 times more potent than vitamin E in its antioxidant capacity, and more effective than vitamin A at protecting cells.

Eye benefits: C, L, O, R

Green or purple seaweed, such as nori, provides high concentrations of vitamin B12, necessary for optimal nerve function. Seaweed also contains omega-3 fatty acids, vital for retinal photoreceptors' structural health and in preventing dry eye and meibomian gland dysfunction.

T

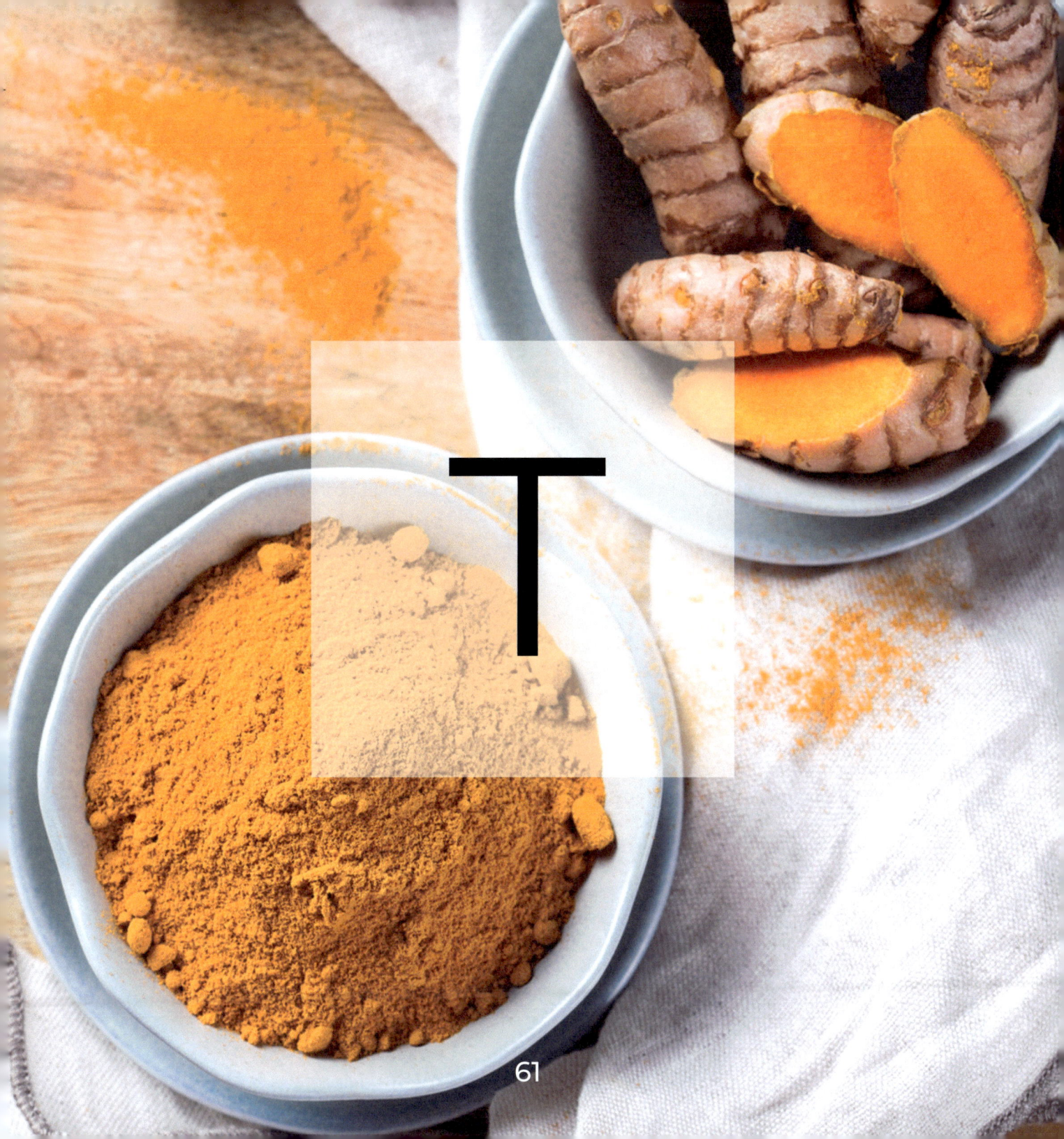

tomato

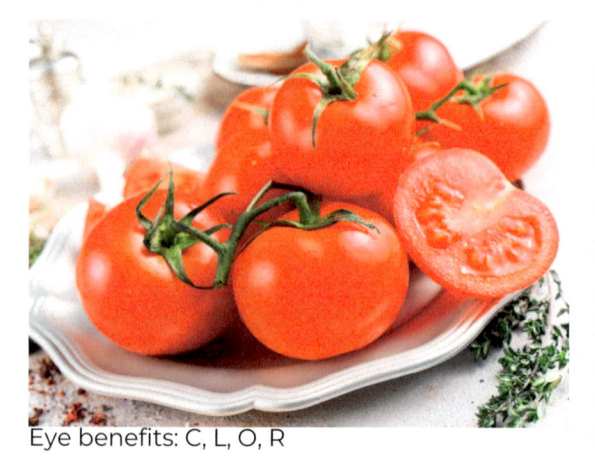

Tomato is a popular fruit that belongs to the nightshade family. It is rich in several key eye health nutrients, such as vitamin C, folate (B9), vitamin K, and potassium.

Tomato is a rich source of several carotenoids, such as lycopene, beta carotene, naringenin, and chlorogenic acid. Lycopene is a pigmented compound that gives the tomato its bright red color. Lycopene and naringenin act as antioxidants with potent anti-inflammatory properties that may help prevent inflammatory eye conditions.

Eye benefits: C, L, O, R

Tomato is 95% water, making it an extremely hydrating fruit. Finally, tomato is an excellent source of insoluble fiber, thus aiding in healthy digestion and waste removal.

turmeric

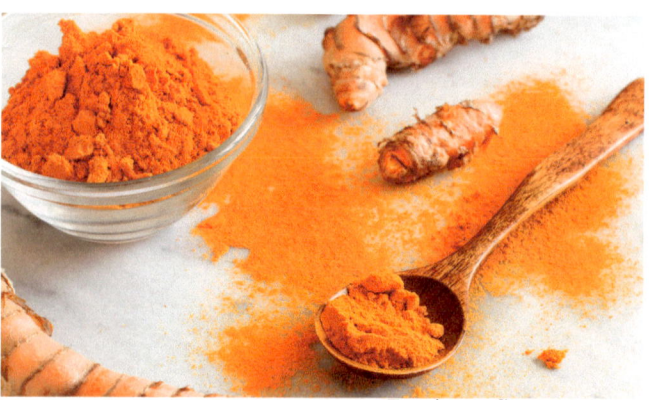

Turmeric is the root (rhizome) of the *Curcumin longa* plant. Curcumin is the active compound in turmeric and can be extracted as a bright yellow spice.

Curcumin is one of the most potent natural anti-inflammatory compounds known to humans. It has shown benefits in many chronic conditions, such as rheumatoid arthritis, diabetes, heart disease, liver disease, and atherosclerosis.

Eye benefits: C, L, O, R

Curcumin from turmeric has been shown in preclinical and clinical studies to benefit a wide range of ocular conditions. These include glaucoma, cataract, age-related macular degeneration, diabetic retinopathy, corneal wound healing, corneal neovascularization, dry eye disease, conjunctivitis, pterygium, and anterior uveitis.

Ugli fruit

Eye benefits: C, L, O, R

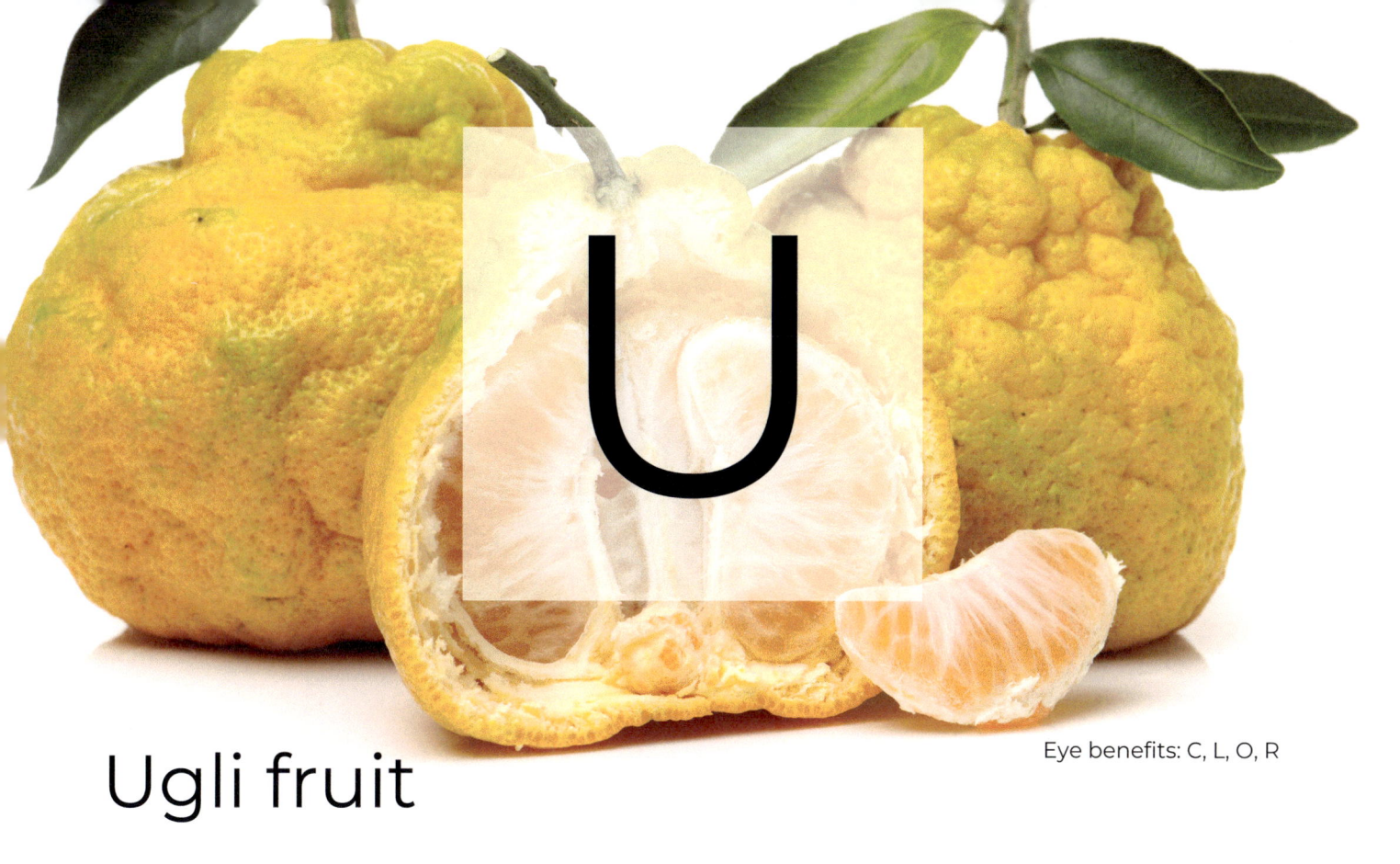

Ugli fruit, also known as Jamaican tangelo, is a cross between a grapefruit and a mandarin orange. It has a thick greenish-yellow skin and a sweet, tangy taste with a hint of bitterness.

Ugli fruit contains a high concentration of vitamin C, 90% of the recommended daily intake. Vitamin C serves as an antioxidant in the fight against cataracts and macular degeneration by preventing damage caused by free radicals. Vitamin C also boosts the immune system to fight against infections and is beneficial for collagen production for the eye's structural support.

Ugli fruit has antioxidant flavonoids, one of which is naringenin. Naringenin has been shown to decrease inflammatory pathways and may be helpful in certain inflammatory eye diseases.

Ugli fruit is low in sugar, making it a good option to help control type 2 diabetes and prevent diabetic retinopathy. The fruit also provides folate (B9), calcium, and potassium which are critical for healthy metabolism and function of the eye muscles.

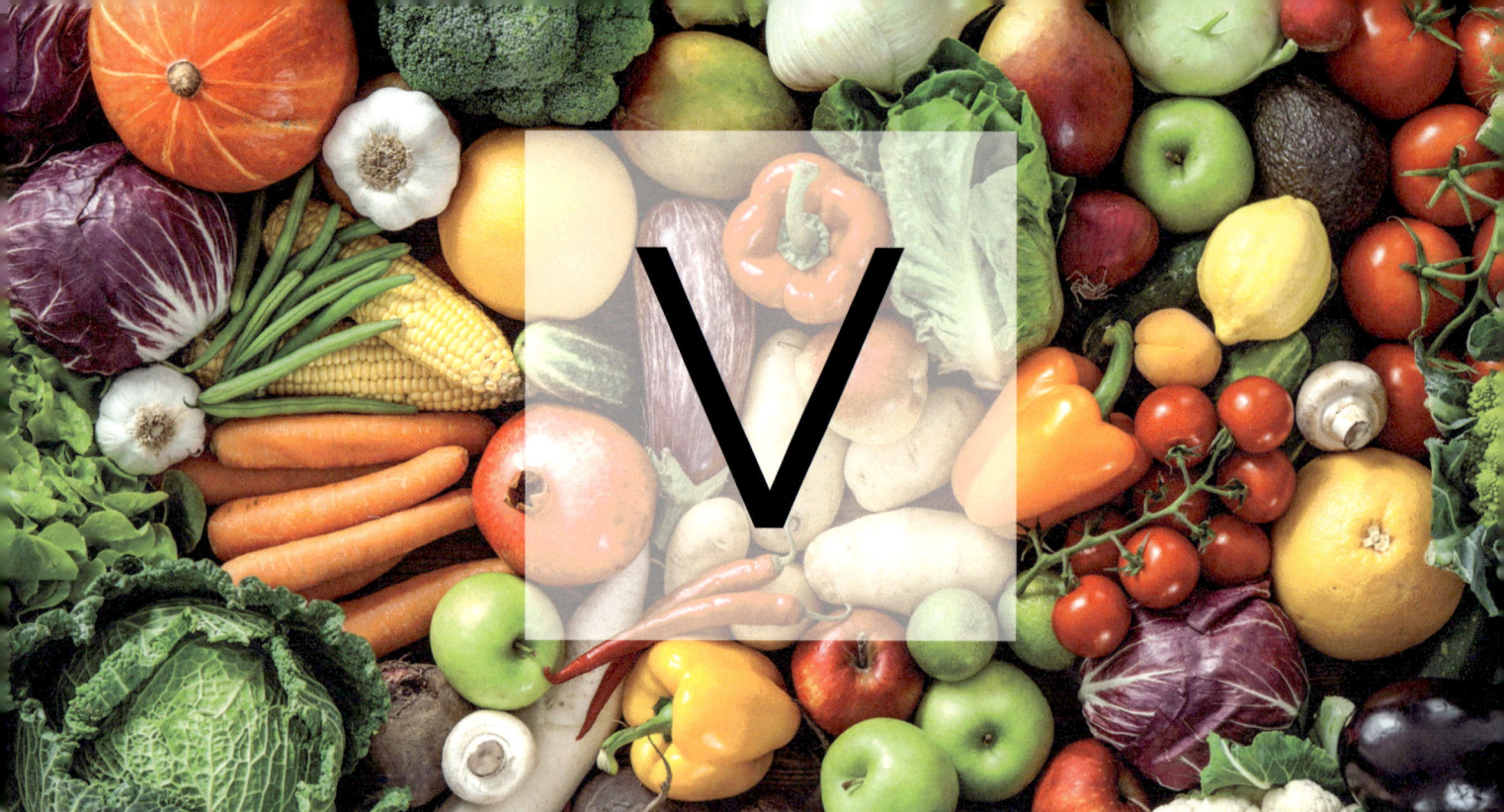

Eye benefits: C, L, O, R

vegetable

You may have noted that many foods highlighted throughout this book are vegetables. The cornerstone of supporting healthy vision is a plant-rich diet, mainly comprised of vegetables.

Rather than eat the same vegetables every day (like carrots) or have only 2 to 3 types of produce every week, it is important that you rotate through your veggies.

It is best to eat a diversity of vegetables from different classes. This will provide your eyes with the full spectrum of vitamins, minerals, and polyphenols they need to stay healthy and fight against many common eye conditions.

For example, the cruciferous, leafy greens, stem, tuber, and root vegetables each have unique benefits and nutrient profiles, so be sure to include several vegetables from each group during the week.

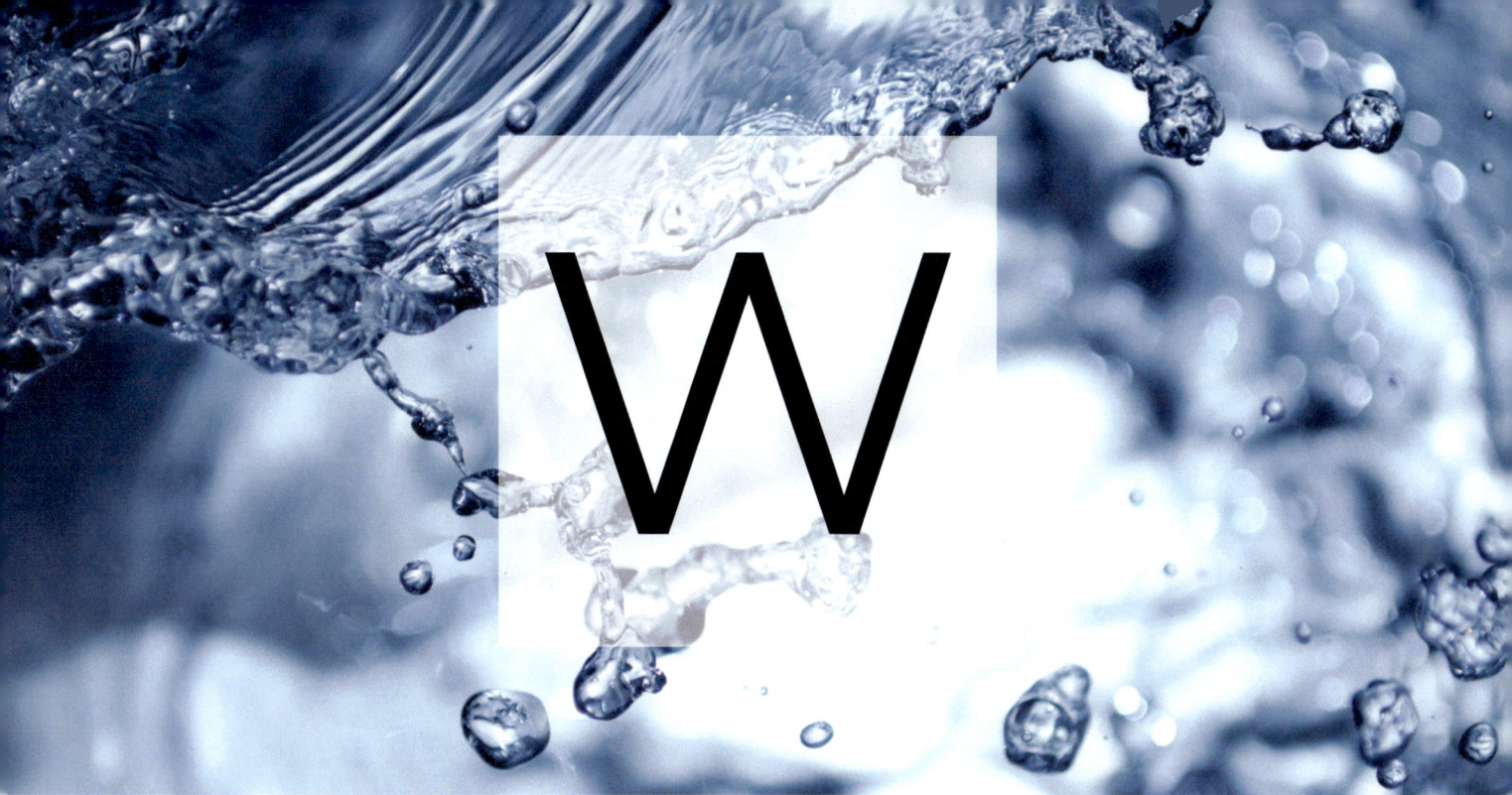

water

Eye benefits: C, L, O, R

Water is the key to good health. Without hydration, your cells cannot function normally. You cannot convert food into energy, deliver oxygen and nutrients via circulation to the delicate tissues of your eyes, maintain structural support of your eye tissues, remove waste products, and detoxify. Hydration is also key to preventing an eye stroke that can affect your optic nerve.

There are two general rules of thumb to determine your hydration requirements:
1. Take your weight in pounds and divide by two for the fluid ounces you should drink daily.
2. The color of your urine should be a light straw color. If it's dark yellow, amber, or orange color, you may be dehydrated.

Hydration guidelines should be adjusted for medical conditions such as your heart and kidney status. Be sure to check with your doctor before determining your hydration needs. Keep in mind that hydration does not only mean drinking water. Other liquids such as coconut water can help you meet your hydration needs. Many fruits and vegetables contain high concentrations of water. Thus, it may be just as important to eat and not only drink your water.

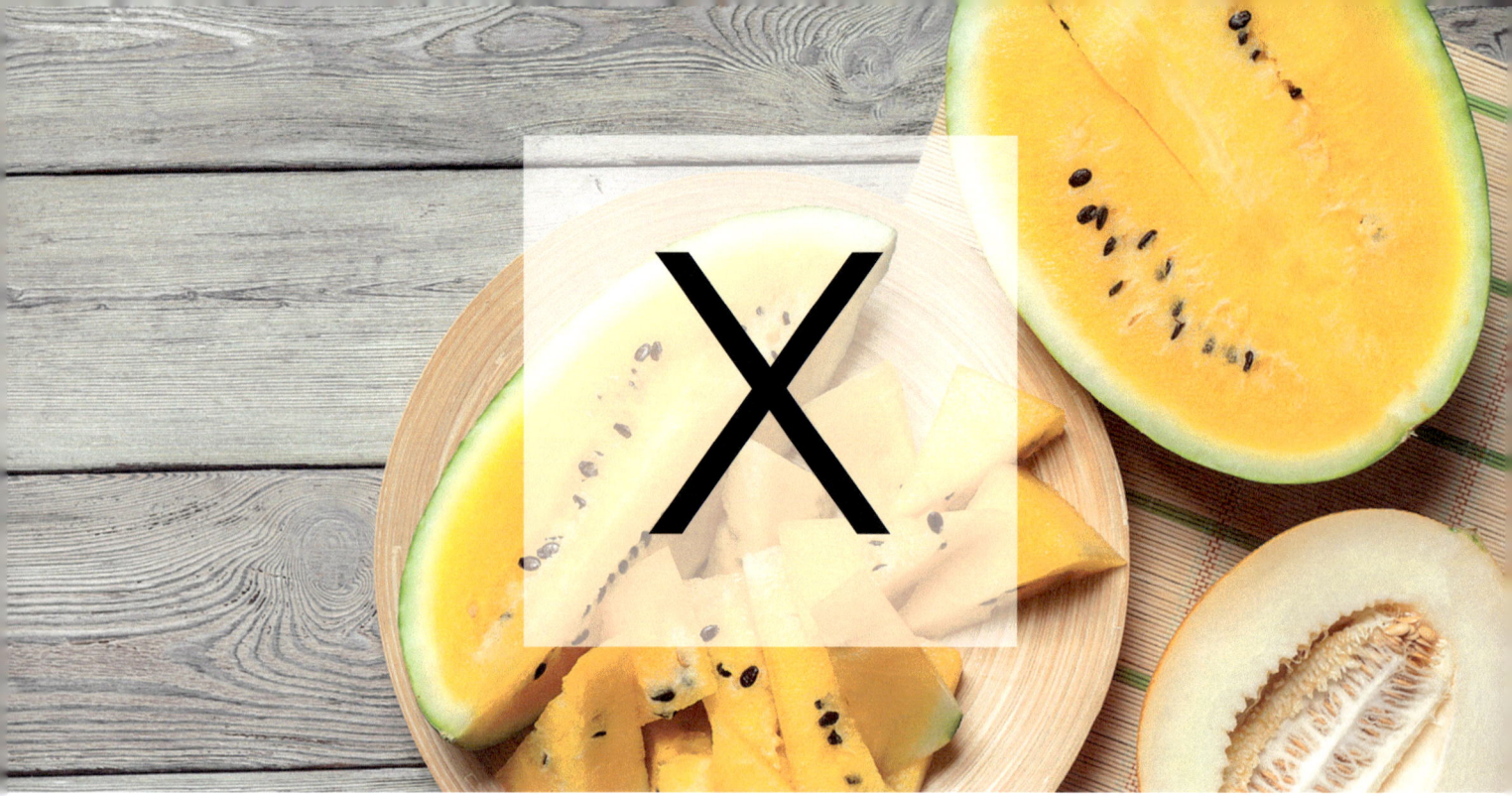

Xigua watermelon

Eye benefits: C, L, O, R

Xigua (pronounced "she- gwah") is a type of watermelon related to fruits like squash, pumpkin, cantaloupe, and cucumber. Originating from Africa, Xigua can be found worldwide and is now commonly cultivated in China.

Xigua watermelon has many nutrients beneficial for eye health. These include vitamins A and C, lycopene, and potassium.

Xigua provides a phytonutrient called citrulline, which is converted into L-arginine, an amino acid. L-arginine helps improve circulation by boosting nitric oxide levels by dilating blood vessels and improving blood flow. Thus, citrulline from Xigua helps to provide oxygen and other nutrients to meet the high metabolic demands of your eye.

Finally, another important health benefit of Xigua is that it contains a high-water concentration and is a hydrating fruit.

Eye benefits: C, L, O, R

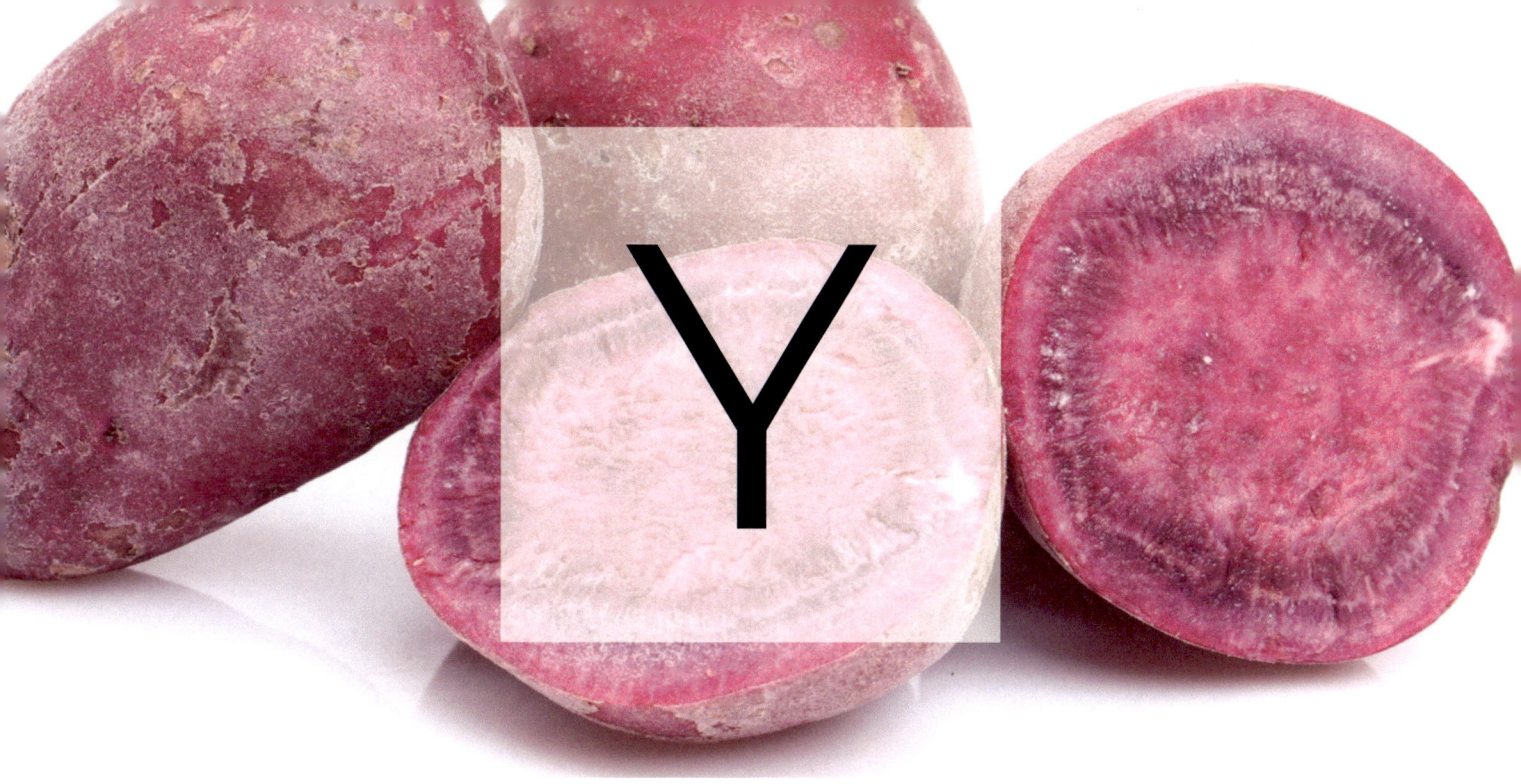

yam

Often mistaken for sweet potato, yam is more starchy and less sweet. Yam has an exterior bark-like skin. Its interior may come in yellow, purple, pink, or white. Yam is nutrient-dense and provides thiamine (B1), pantothenic acid (B5), folate (B9), vitamins A and C, magnesium, potassium, copper, and manganese. Yam also contains a unique compound called diosgenin. In early clinical studies of cognitive function, diosgenin has been shown to improve nerve cell health and brain function.

Ube, also known as purple or violet yam, has additional eye health benefits. Ube contains pigmented antioxidants called anthocyanins that provide its beautiful purple and violet hues. Anthocyanins such as cyanidin-3-glucoside have protective benefits against oxidative stress, the root cause of age-related eye diseases, such as glaucoma, cataract, and macular degeneration.

Though a starchy vegetable, yam has a low glycemic index of 24, reducing blood sugar spikes and improving glycemic control. Finally, yam is a prebiotic food that is an abundant source of soluble and insoluble fiber, important for digestion and gut health. Yam has been shown to promote the growth of healthy gut bacteria like Bifidobacterium and Lactobacillus species.

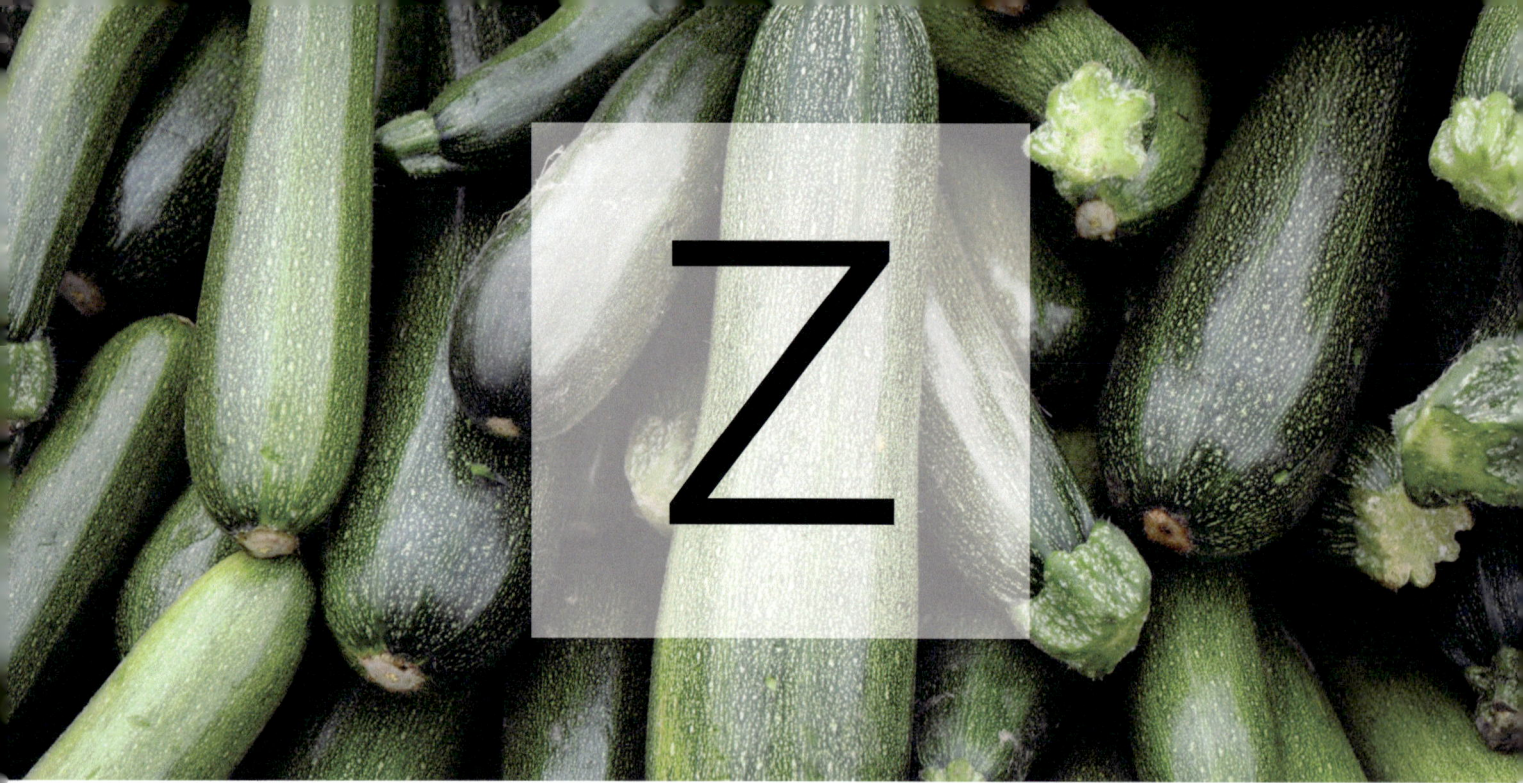

Eye benefits: C, L, O, R

zucchini

Last but certainly not least in the alphabet of foods for eye health is zucchini. Also known as courgette, zucchini is a member of the summer squash family, cousin to cucumber, spaghetti squash, and melon.

Zucchini is an excellent source of many eye health nutrients- vitamins A, C, and K, thiamine (B1), folate (B9), and pyridoxine (B6). Zucchini provides a host of minerals to ensure healthy metabolism and energy production – magnesium, manganese, potassium, copper, and phosphorus.

Zucchini contains carotenoid antioxidants- lutein, zeaxanthin, and beta carotene- important for retinal health to fight against night blindness and macular degeneration.

Zucchini is an excellent source of water, essential for proper digestion and detoxification. Finally, zucchini supplies soluble and insoluble fiber; soluble fiber helps feed your gut microbiome, and insoluble fiber promotes healthy digestion by adding bulk to stools.

Part III

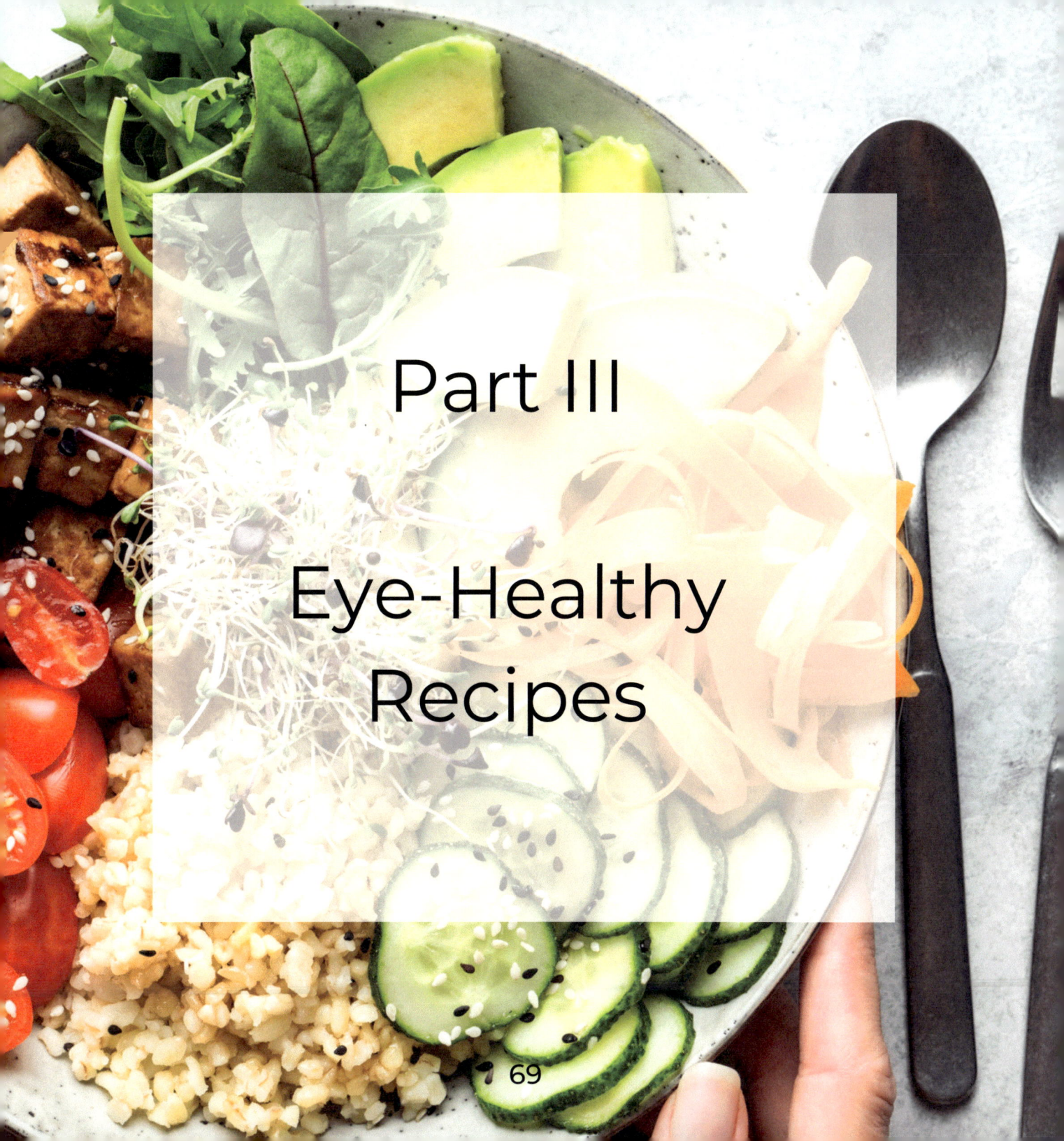

Eye-Healthy Recipes

blueberry avocado spinach smoothie

Ingredients:

½ cup unsweetened vanilla almond milk
½ ripe avocado
1 cup spinach
1 medium ripe banana
2 cups frozen blueberries
1 tbsp whole almonds
1 tbsp ground flaxseed meal
¼ tsp cinnamon
fresh mint leaves

Directions:

Put all ingredients in the blender in order starting with almond milk, spinach, banana, avocado, blueberries, flaxseed meal, and almonds.

Blend until smooth and add a handful of ice for a thicker smoothie. Garnish with mint.

Serves 1-2.

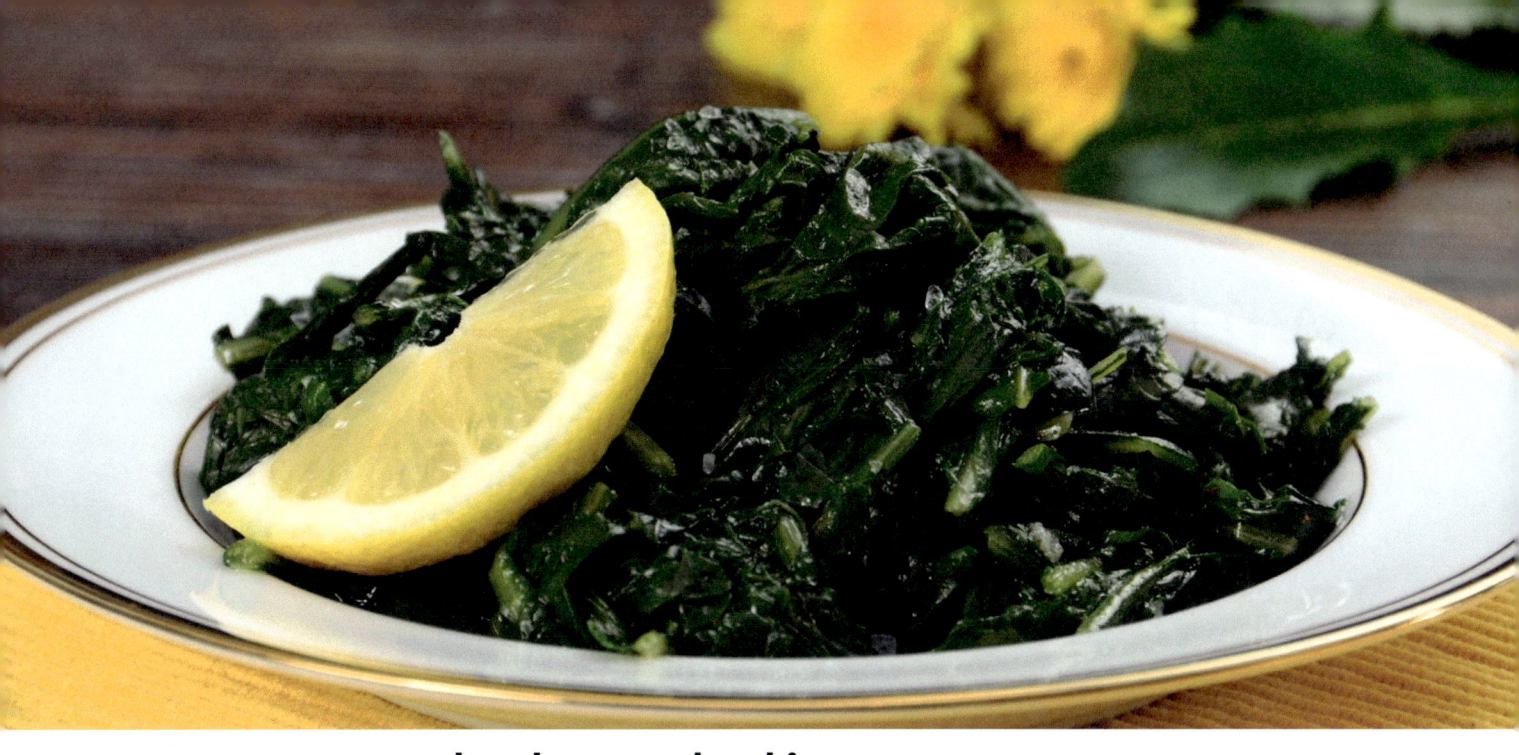

sauteed dandelion greens

Ingredients

1 bunch dandelion greens
2 tbsps extra-virgin olive oil
4 large garlic cloves
Pinch of red pepper flakes
Celtic sea salt to taste
Lemon for garnish

Serves 2-4.

Directions

Trim off and discard the bottom one to two inches of the thick stems. To clean them, submerge them in a bowl of cold water. Make 2-inch-long portions. Greens from dandelion plants are added to a large pot of boiling, salted water.

Cook uncovered for 10 minutes until tender. They are prepared when the stem of a dandelion green can be pierced with a fork. Water should be drained, cooled, and squeezed out. In a sauté pan, heat olive oil over medium-low heat. Red pepper flakes and garlic may be added; sauté for 30 seconds or until just beginning to turn golden.

Add dandelion greens and sea salt. Turn up the heat to medium, then sauté for 5 minutes or until tender. Add lemon for garnish.

multi-greens smoothie with green tea

Ingredients:

1 cup kale, collards, or Swiss chard, packed tight (large stems removed)
½ cup loosely packed parsley leaves
1 medium apple, cored
1 medium pear, cored
1 tablespoon lemon or lime juice
1 cup green tea, cold or room temp
½ cup water
¾ cup ice

Directions

Put all ingredients in a high-power blender, and start on low speed, gradually working up to high speed for 1 minute.

Tips: This is best if served fresh, but it may be stored in the refrigerator to drink later in the day if desired. Try to use a variety of different greens each time the Multi-Greens Smoothie is prepared if used daily or frequently. If controlling carbohydrates more tightly, cut fruit portions in half.

Serves 2.

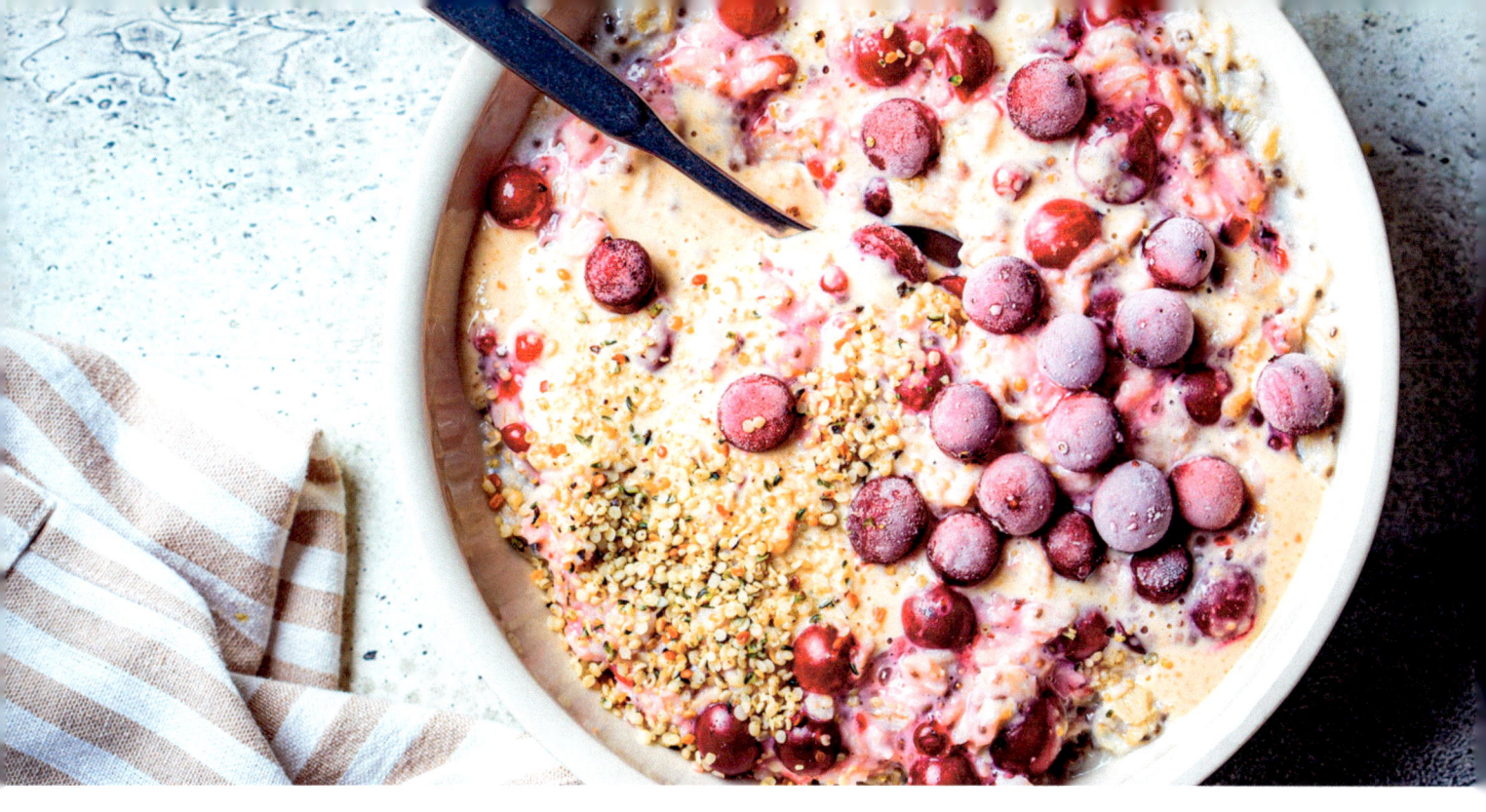

hemp, chia, and flax oatmeal

Ingredients

1 cup raw hemp seeds
2 tbsps. chia seeds
2 tbsps. flaxseed meal
2 cups almond milk (or other non-dairy milk)
1 cup cranberries, strawberries, or berries of choice
¼ cup slivered almonds (optional)
4 tbsps. natural sweetener of choice
Pinch of salt

Directions

In a pot, combine hemp seeds, chia seeds, flaxseed meal, almond milk, natural sweetener, and salt. Over medium heat, stir continuously for approximately 4 mins.

Remove from heat and top with berries and almonds (optional)

Serves 2.

strawberry peach kale smoothie

Ingredients

2 cups unsweetened almond, hemp, or coconut milk
1 cup frozen strawberries (no sugar added)
1 cup frozen peaches (no sugar added)
2 cups fresh organic kale
1 tablespoon ground flax or chia seeds
1 teaspoon vanilla extract
2 scoops vanilla protein powder

Directions

Put all in a blender and mix well. Add ice to make smoothie slushier, if desired.

Tips: May substitute organic baby spinach for the kale.

Serves 2.

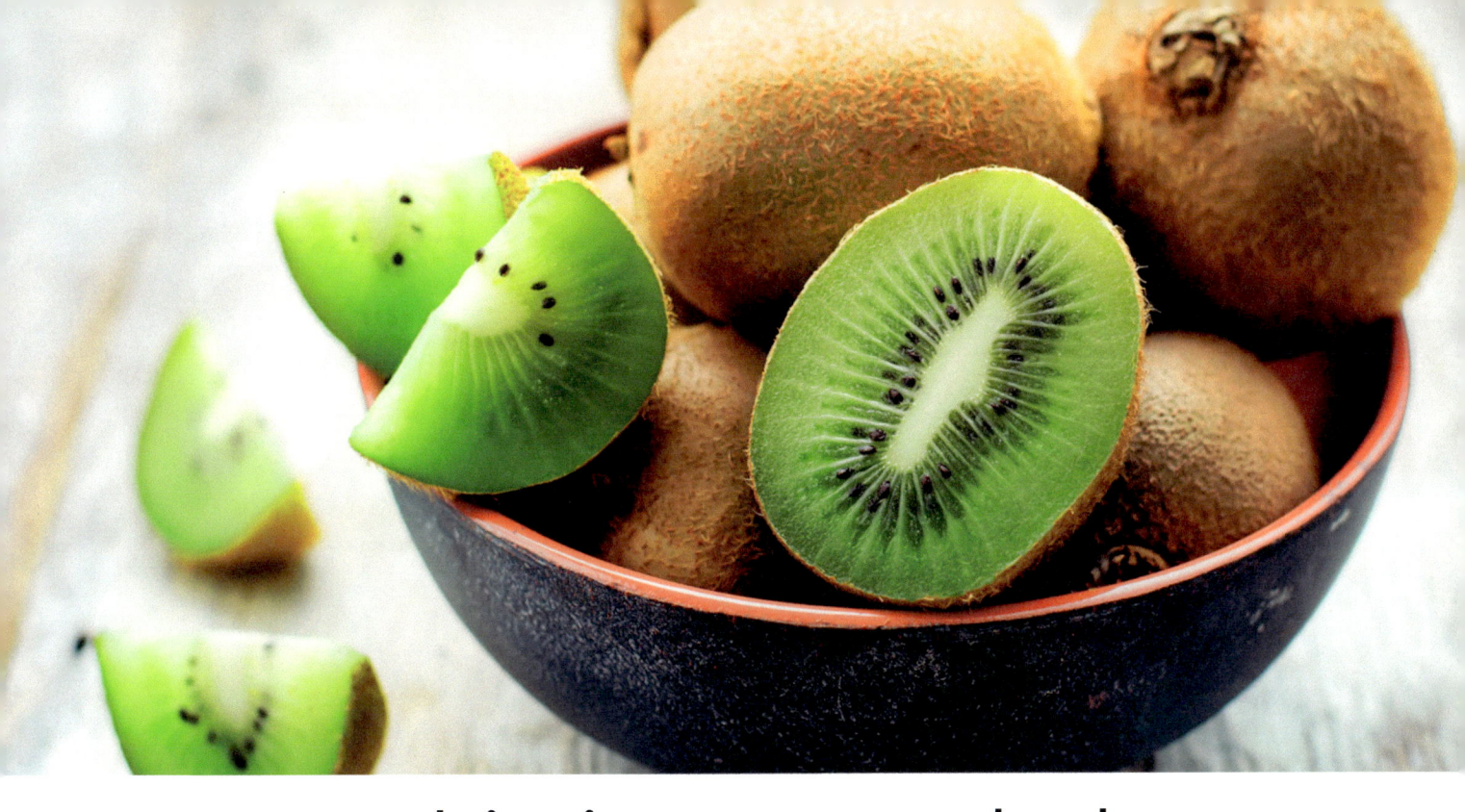

orange kiwi green salad

Ingredients

6 cups mixed greens
2 kiwis, peeled and sliced
2-3 Mandarin oranges, peeled
2-3 red onions, thinly sliced

Directions

Rinse mixed greens and dry. On a serving plate, add mixed greens. Next add kiwi, mandarin oranges, and onions.

Serves 4.

watermelon nectarine and mint cooler

Ingredients

4-5 cups seedless watermelon chunks
2 nectarines, peeled and sliced
1 ½ cups seltzer water
Fresh mint sprigs
1-2 tbsps. natural sweetener

Directions

In a blender, add watermelon and nectarine chucks. Blend until liquid.

Add seltzer water and natural sweetener to taste.

Pour over ice and top with fresh mint.

Serves 4.

mushroom and bell pepper sauté with greens

Ingredients

3 tbsps. olive oil, divided
½ pound cremini mushrooms, cut in half, or 2 medium portabellas, thinly sliced
1 large bell pepper (red, orange, or yellow), sliced very thin
2 cloves garlic, minced
¼ cup chopped fresh basil leaves (or 1 tbsp dried)
1 tbsp balsamic vinegar
1 tbsp lemon juice
4 cups mixed greens

Directions

Heat 2 tbsps. olive oil over medium heat in a large skillet.
Add mushrooms and bell peppers, and sauté until tender, about 7-10 mins.
Add garlic, and sauté for 1 more min.
Stir in the fresh or dried basil, balsamic vinegar, and lemon juice, cooking over low heat until liquid is reduced by half, about 2 mins.
Divide greens among 4 plates, and drizzle with the remaining 1 tbsp olive oil. Top with warm peppers and mushrooms and serve immediately.

Serves 4.

quinoa with corn, cashews, and black beans

Ingredients

1 cup quinoa, rinsed
1 ½ cup black beans, drained, rinsed, and cooked
1 cup cooked sweet corn
2 cups water
½ cup Inca berries (optional)
1/2 cup tomato, diced
½ cup cashews, chopped
¼ cup cilantro, chopped
2 cloves garlic, minced
2 tbsps. coconut oil
1 tsp caraway seeds
½ tsp salt

Directions

Over medium heat, cook garlic and caraway seeds in 1 tbsp coconut oil. Add quinoa, water, and salt. Bring to a boil and reduce to a simmer for 10-15mins. Add in the black beans and 1 tbsp coconut oil and cook for another 10-15 mins.

In another pan over medium heat, toast the cashews.

In the quinoa pot, add the corn, tomato, half the cashews, and half the coriander. Serve and top with Inca berries (optional) and the rest of the cashews and coriander.

Serves 4.

Jerusalem artichoke soup with cabbage and rosemary

Ingredients

1 tbsp extra virgin olive oil
2.12 oz onion
3.53 oz leek, chopped
1 garlic clove, chopped
1 tbsp dill
1 tsp thyme
4.23 oz cabbage, shredded
2.82 oz carrots, peeled and chopped
2.12 oz Jerusalem artichoke
2 cups water
rosemary sprigs
Salt to taste
Black pepper to taste

Directions

In a pan over medium heat, add olive oil and cook onion until golden brown. Add garlic, thyme, leek, and dill, and cook for 3 mins.

Next, add Jerusalem artichokes, carrots, and cabbage and cook for 5 mins. Add water and simmer for 10mins until carrots are cooked.

Remove from heat and blend with a hand blender until you get a creamy, velvety consistency. Add salt and black pepper to taste. Garnish with fresh rosemary sprigs.

Serves 2.

peppermint green tea

Ingredients

4 bags organic green tea
4 bags peppermint tea
12 cups water, divided

Directions

Fill a glass coffee pot with 8 cups of water and add to the coffee maker.

Place the 8 tea bags in the filter section of the coffee maker. Turn on the coffee maker, and let it run through a cycle.

Pour the tea concentrate into a large pitcher, add 4 cups of cool water, and serve.

Tip: Tea will stay fresh in the refrigerator for 5–7 days.

Serves 12 (1 serving = 1 cup/8 fluid ounces).

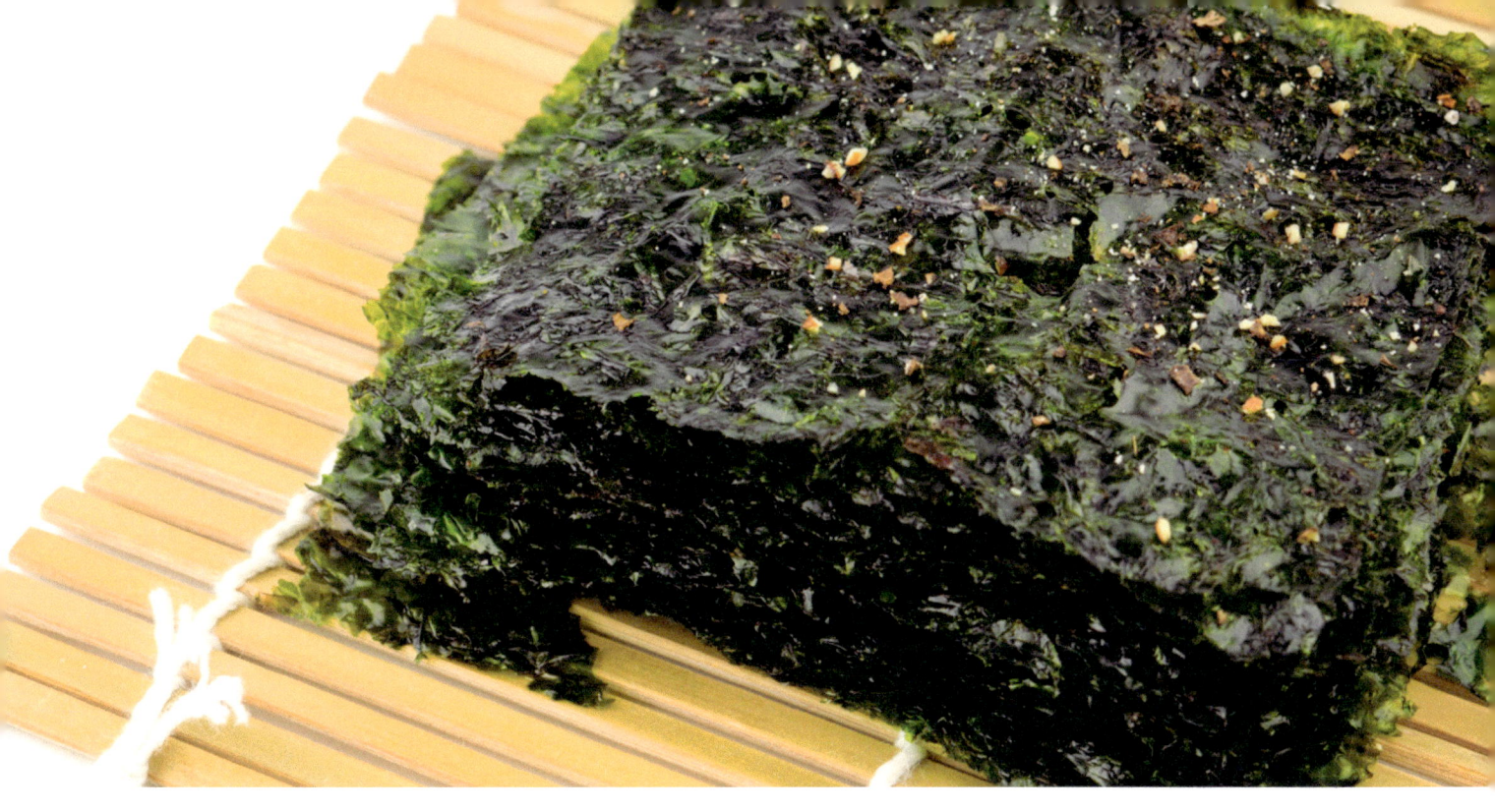

bulgar roasted seaweed rolls

Ingredients

2 cups water
1 cup bulgur
½ tsp sea salt
2 tbsps. rice vinegar
½ tsp sugar
½ tsp sesame seed oil
Nori sheets (roasted seaweed), cut in half
1 medium carrot, shredded (about 1 cup)
1 medium cucumber, seeded, cut into thin strips

Directions

Bring water to a boil in a medium pan. Add salt and bulgur and stir. Remove from heat and let it sit for 25 mins. Drain excess water and set it aside.

Next, stir the rice vinegar, sugar, and sesame seed oil into the bulgur. Add 2 tbsps of bulgur into the center of each nori sheet.

Then, add cucumber and carrots on top. Fold the nori sheet from the corners towards the center into a cone.

Serves 4.

roasted vegetables with thyme and rosemary

Ingredients

1 butternut squash, peeled and cubed
1-2 zucchini, sliced
1-2 yellow squash, sliced
1 cup white button mushrooms
3 bell peppers- red, orange, and yellow
½ cup low sodium broth
1 tsp dried rosemary
1 tsp dried thyme
Dash of pepper
Sprinkle of Himalayan salt

Directions

Preheat the oven to 425 degrees F.

Place parchment paper on a baking sheet. In a large bowl, add all the vegetables, broth, rosemary, thyme, salt, and pepper, and mix.

Place vegetables on the baking sheet and roast for 35-40mins until soft and tender.

Mix vegetables halfway through cooking time and add more broth if needed.

Serves 6-7.

three bean vegetable chili

Ingredients

1 tablespoon olive oil
½ large onion, diced
2 carrots, diced
1 red bell pepper, chopped
1 clove garlic, finely chopped
1 jalapeno pepper, seeded and minced
1 ½ tablespoons chili powder
2 teaspoons ground cumin
1 ½ teaspoons dried oregano
1 can (28 ounces) no-salt added diced tomatoes
1 cup water
1 can (15 ounces) black beans, rinsed and drained
1 can (15 ounces) red kidney beans, rinsed and drained
1 can (15 ounces) Great Northern beans, rinsed and drained
½ teaspoon sea salt

Garnish
Fresh cilantro
Chopped scallions

Directions

Heat oil in large saucepan or stockpot. Add onions, carrots, bell peppers, garlic, and jalapeno and cook until onion is translucent (about 5 minutes).
Add dry spices (chili powder, cumin, and oregano), and cook for a 1 minute, stirring frequently.
Add canned tomatoes including juices, water, beans, and salt. Bring to boil, reduce heat, and then simmer uncovered for 30 minutes.
Serve garnished with chopped cilantro and scallions.

Tips

Try to find low-sodium canned beans. Otherwise, be sure to rinse beans well after draining to reduce sodium.

Serves 6.

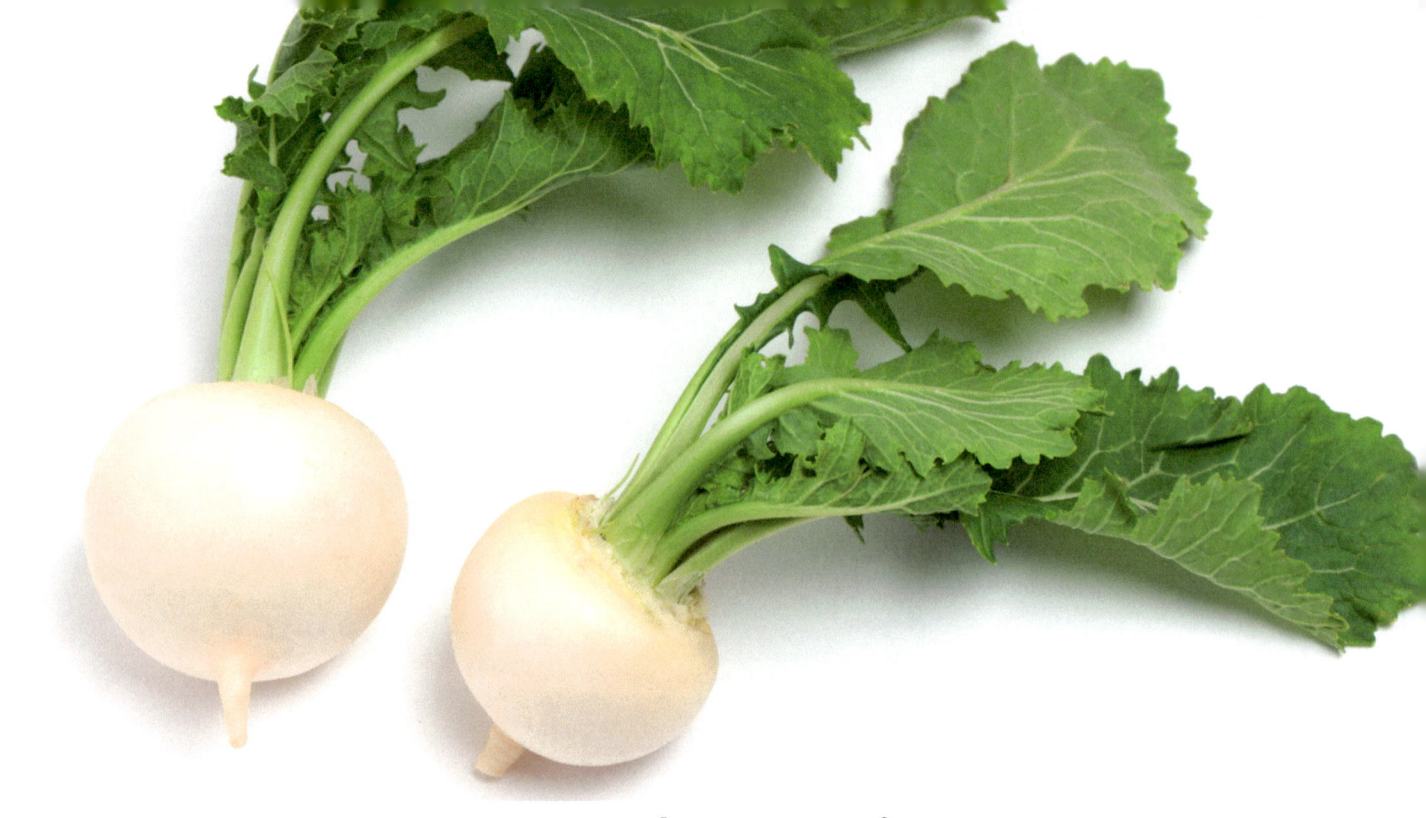

sweet corn and turnip greens

Ingredients

1 tbsp olive oil
½ cup onion, chopped
2 cloves garlic, mashed
3 cups turnip greens, washed, drained, coarsely chopped
2 cups water
3 cups fresh sweet corn
2 Roma tomatoes, seeded and chopped
½ tsp red pepper flakes
1 tsp balsamic vinegar
Salt and black pepper to taste

Serves 6.

Directions

In a pan over medium heat, heat olive oil. Add the onions and cook until translucent. Add the garlic and cook until fragrant.

Add turnip greens and quickly toss. Next, add the water and bring it to a boil. Simmer for about 15 mins. Add corn and bring to a boil.

Next, add the tomatoes, red pepper flakes, and balsamic vinegar. Cook for about 5 mins until greens are tender and corn is firm. Add salt and pepper.

baked yams with aioli

Ingredients

6 yams
¾ cup extra virgin olive oil (EVOO)
½ cup grapeseed oil
2 whole cloves garlic, plus ½ clove, grated
Pinch of saffron threads, crushed
1 cup raw cashews
3/4 cup water
2 – 4 garlic cloves
2 teaspoons Dijon mustard
juice of 1/2 lemon
pinch of mineral salt, or to taste

Directions

Preheat oven to 400 degrees F. Score each yam with a knife and place on a baking sheet. Bake for 45 mins.

In a pan, cook EVOO, grapeseed oil, garlic, and saffron over medium-low heat for about 15 mins. Remove garlic from the pan and mash with salt. Set aside.

Prepare the aioli: Place cashews, water, garlic, Dijon, and juice of lemon in a blender and blend until creamy, about 45 seconds. Taste for flavor, adding a little more of desired ingredients to taste. Serve at room temperature. Refrigerate in an airtight container for up to a week.

Remove the yams from the oven and slightly cool. Split the yams open and top with aioli. Sprinkle with parsley or herbs of your choice.

Serves 6.

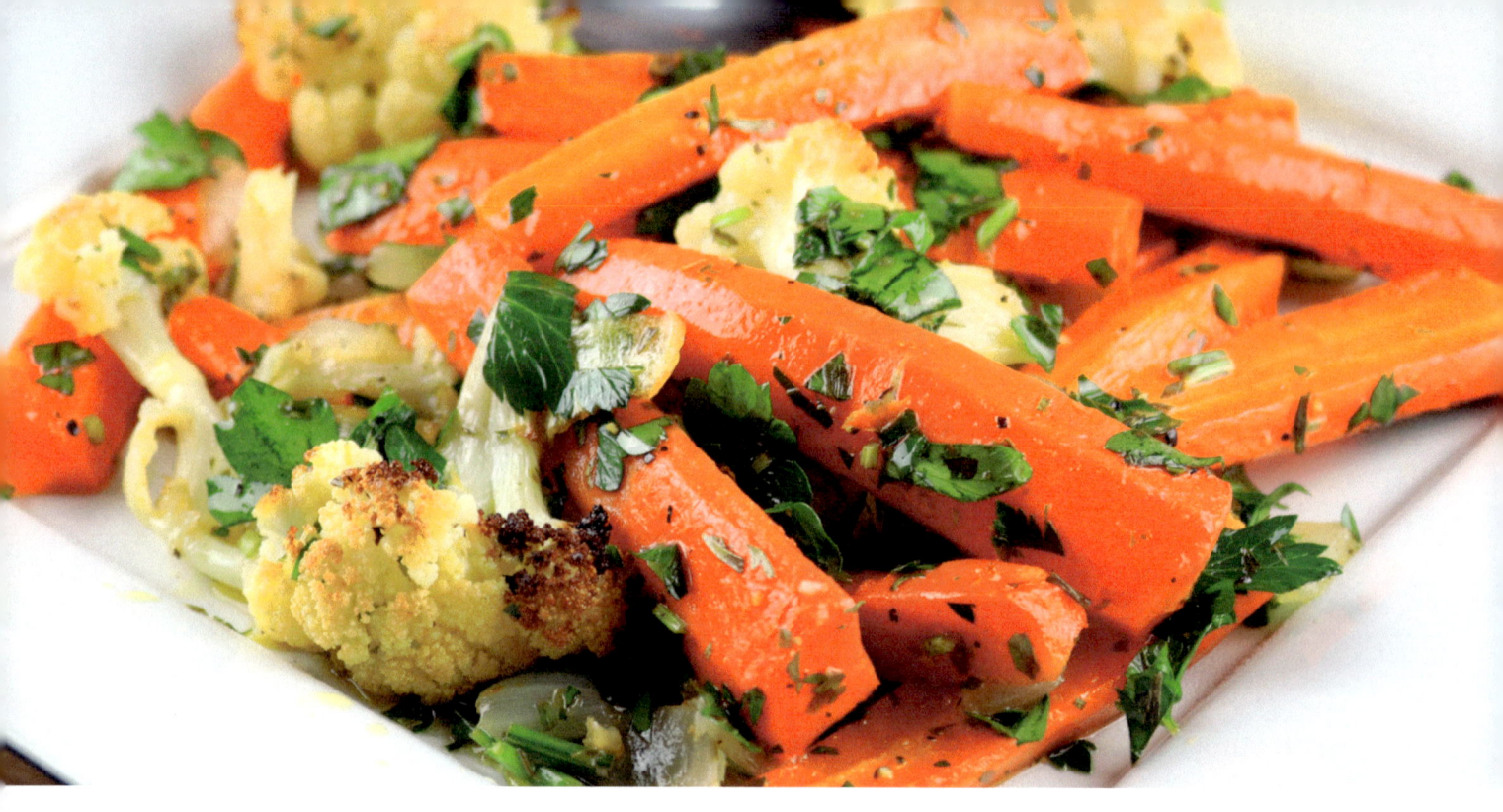

roasted cauliflower with carrots

Ingredients

1 small head cauliflower chopped into small florets
4 medium carrots, peeled and sliced
2 tbsps. parsley, chopped
¼ tsp turmeric
¼ tsp dried thyme
½ tsp grated lemon zest
4 tsp extra virgin olive oil
Salt and ground black pepper

Serves 4.

Directions

Preheat the oven to 450 degrees F. On a baking sheet, toss the cauliflower and carrots in 3 tsp. of olive oil, thyme, ½ tsp salt, 1/4 tsp turmeric, and ¼ tsp pepper until coated. Spread the vegetables evenly. Roast the vegetables for 25 mins until lightly browned.

Sprinkle the thyme, lemon zest, and 1 tsp of olive oil over roasted vegetables.

sauteed mustard greens

Ingredients

½ cup red onions, thinly sliced
2 cloves garlic, minced
1 tbsp extra virgin olive oil
1 lb. mustard greens, washed and torn into pieces
2-3 tbsps. vegetable broth
¼ tsp salt
¼ tsp pepper
¼ tsp sesame oil

Directions

In a pan, sauté onions in olive oil for about 5-10 mins until onions caramelize.

Next, cook garlic until fragrant.

Add mustard greens and broth until greens are wilted.

Toss with sesame oil. Sprinkle it with salt and pepper.

Serves 4.

cherry chia seed pudding

Ingredients

½ cup chia seeds
2 tsps. of natural sweetener of choice
2 cups frozen cherries
2 cups unsweetened almond milk
½ cup water

Directions

In a medium bowl, mix chia seeds, almond milk, and natural sweetener. Cover and soak for 4 hours or overnight.

Blend water and frozen cherries until you have a thick sauce. Place sauce in a mason jar and add the chia seed mixture on top.

Garnish with your favorite toppings., i.e., cacao nibs and coconut flakes.

Serves 4.

Part IV

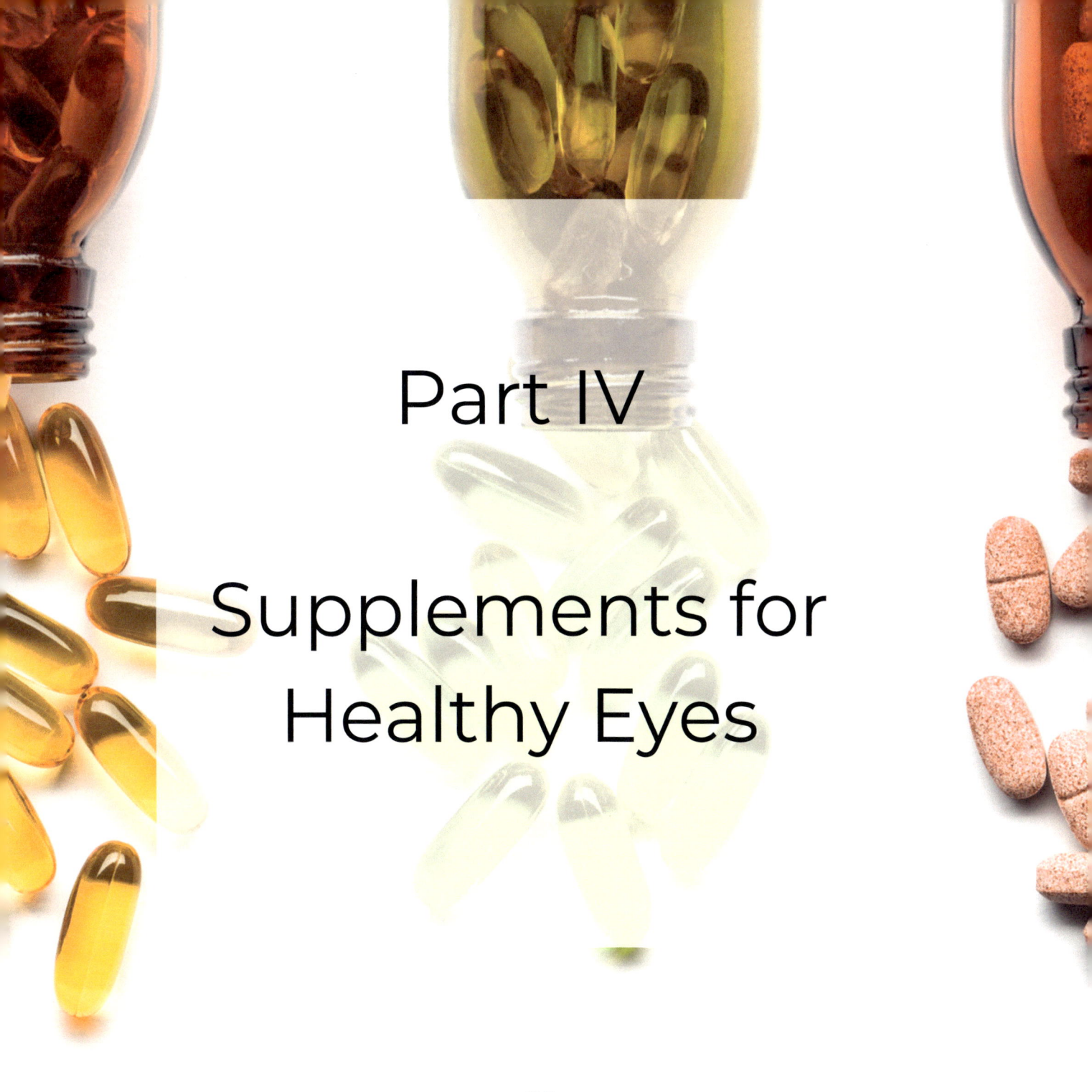

Supplements for Healthy Eyes

Any discussion of the nutrients essential for vision health would not be complete without mentioning supplements for your eyes. In fact, when I counsel my patients about proper nutrition to support their vision, this is one of the first questions that comes up.

My patients often inquire, "Dr. Banik, can all get all the nutrients I need for my eyes from my diet alone, or should I take an eye vitamin? If so, which one? So many are on the shelf, and I don't know which to choose!"

If you've had similar questions about eye vitamins, you are not alone. There are over 75 supplements from various manufacturers on the market touted for eye health! It can be confusing trying to assess which may be best for you.

What is even more challenging is that each supplement brand has its own formulation with unique ingredient profiles and dosages. It may be difficult to assess if you are getting the full support your eyes may need.

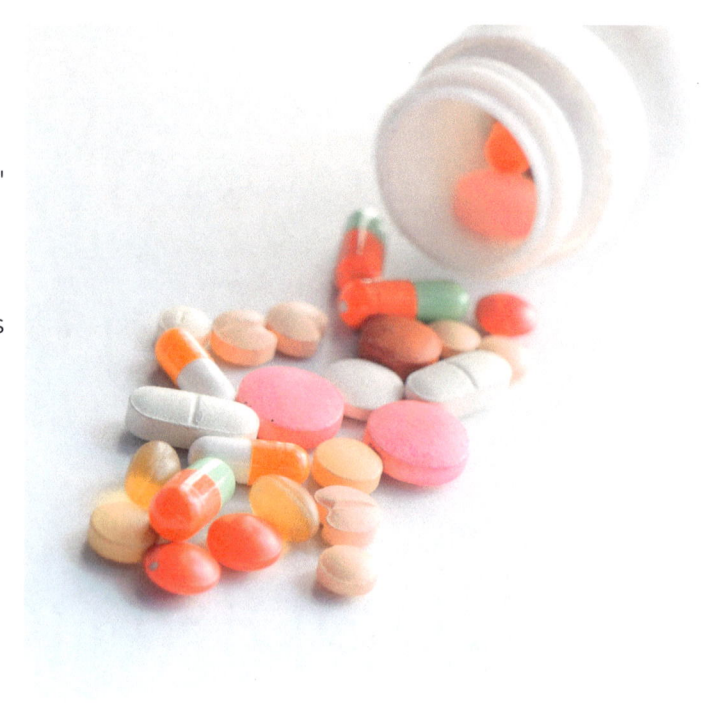

When it comes to eye health supplements, I counsel my patients by stressing two key points -

   1. It is always best to get most of your nutrition from eating a diverse, plant-rich diet. This type of food plan will provide you with the range of vitamins, minerals, and phytonutrients your eyes need to function optimally and prevent disease. Remember that nutrition that comes directly from foods is how nature intended, offering the best absorption or bioavailability.

   2. Unfortunately, most people are not getting the full range of eye nutrients they need from food alone. Therefore, it is prudent for most of us to take a supplement, or better yet, a combination of supplements, to fill in the gaps in our diet and best support our eye health.

The key to these points is that supplements should do exactly that- *supplement* an already healthy, nutrient-rich diet. They should *not* be a substitution for an unhealthy diet.

There are three reasons why eye health supplements are necessary, especially in this day and age. The first is that several of the nutrients essential for vision are difficult to get in sufficient quantities from diet alone.

Let me give you an example. The recommended daily intake of the macular carotenoids, lutein and zeaxanthin, is 6.5 mg and 1-2 mg daily, respectively. The therapeutic foods for eye health (as noted in Part II of this book) that are high in lutein and zeaxanthin include spinach, kale, pistachios, and orange and yellow varieties of bell peppers. However, to get enough of your macular carotenoid requirements, large amounts of these foods would need to be eaten daily,

Studies have shown that unfortunately, people on a Western-style diet get only 1-2 mg of lutein and less than 1 mg of zeaxanthin per day. In comparison, indigenous populations for whom a plant and fiber-rich diet is the norm, such as those living in the Fiji islands, get over 25 mg of lutein daily!

The bottom line is that the standard Western diet simply does not provide enough lutein and zeaxanthin, two critical nutrients to prevent macular degeneration and neutralize any potential damage from UV and blue light.

Thus, supplementation with certain eye health nutrients is a MUST for those of us who want to be proactive in protecting and preserving our delicate macula, responsible for our central vision.

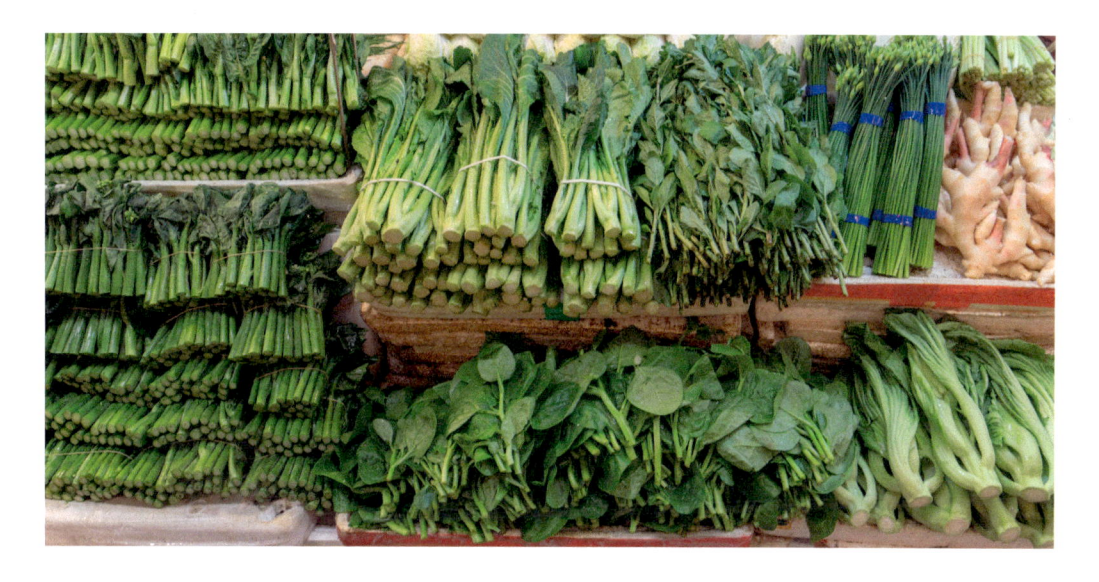

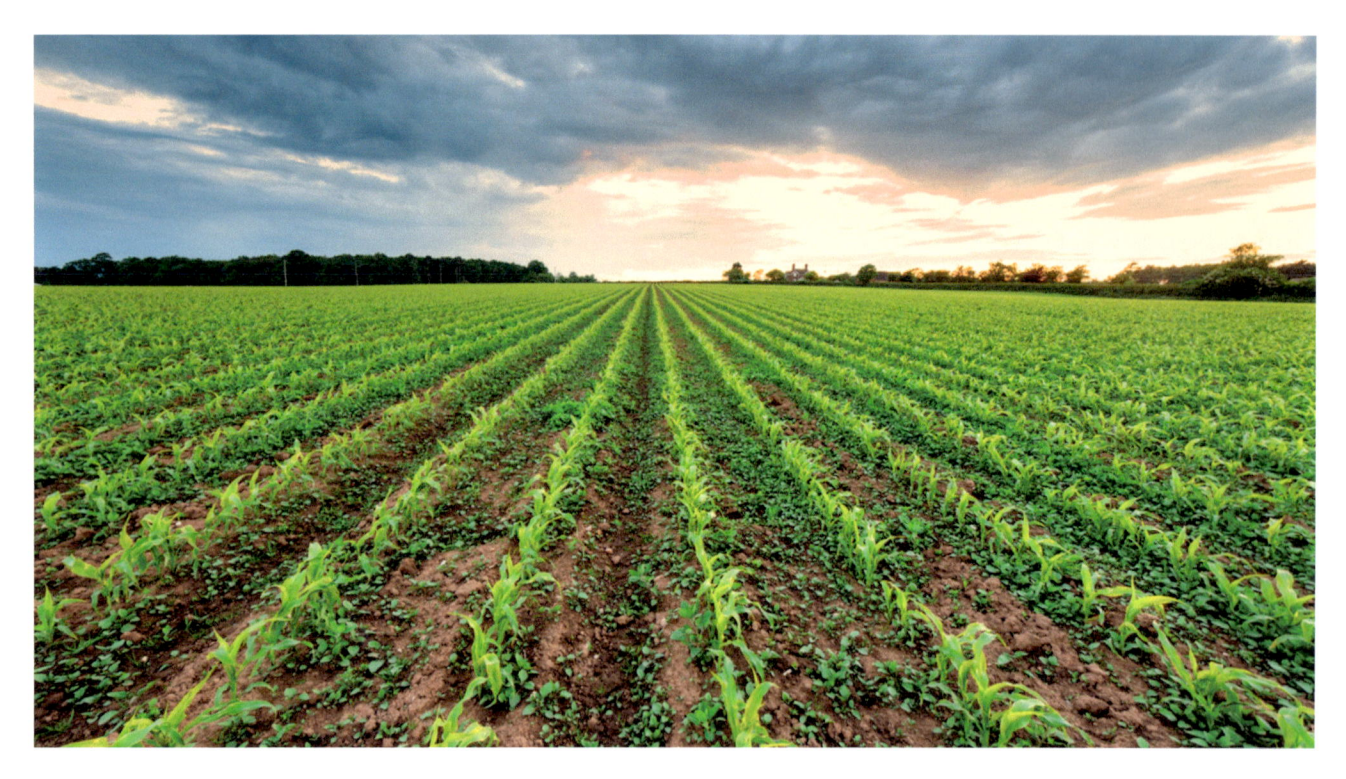

The second unfortunate truth about nutrients and food is that current agricultural practices that have been designed to increase crop yields, such as the use of chemical fertilizers, crop rotation, and tilling, have led to the depletion of nutrients in the soil.

The fact is that food grown today is not as nutritionally dense as it used to be in decades past, such as in the 1930s and 1940s. For example, studies have shown that the use of nitrogen fertilizers can decrease nutrients in crops such as Vitamin C and other phytonutrients.

Another nutrient vital for eye, brain, and overall health is magnesium, a mineral involved in over 600 enzymatic reactions in the body. Over the last fifty years, magnesium levels have been found to be decreased in the soil and subsequently, in fruits and vegetables we eat. To make matters worse, food processing depletes over 80% of this critical mineral necessary for optimal health. Most of us are thus magnesium-deficient.

Because of these inadequacies in the nutritional value of our diet and food, most of which are beyond our control, supplementation is a *necessity* for eye health.

Finally, the third reason why it is prudent to take a dietary supplement to protect and preserve your vision is that our eyes are exposed to environmental stressors as they have never been before.

Light exposure, especially to artificial blue light emitted by all digital screens and energy-saving bulbs, is at an all-time high. We live in a digital world where most adults on average spend over ten hours a day on a screen.

Even children, whose eyes are still developing and potentially more vulnerable to the health-related side effects of blue light exposure, spend at least six hours a day on a screen.

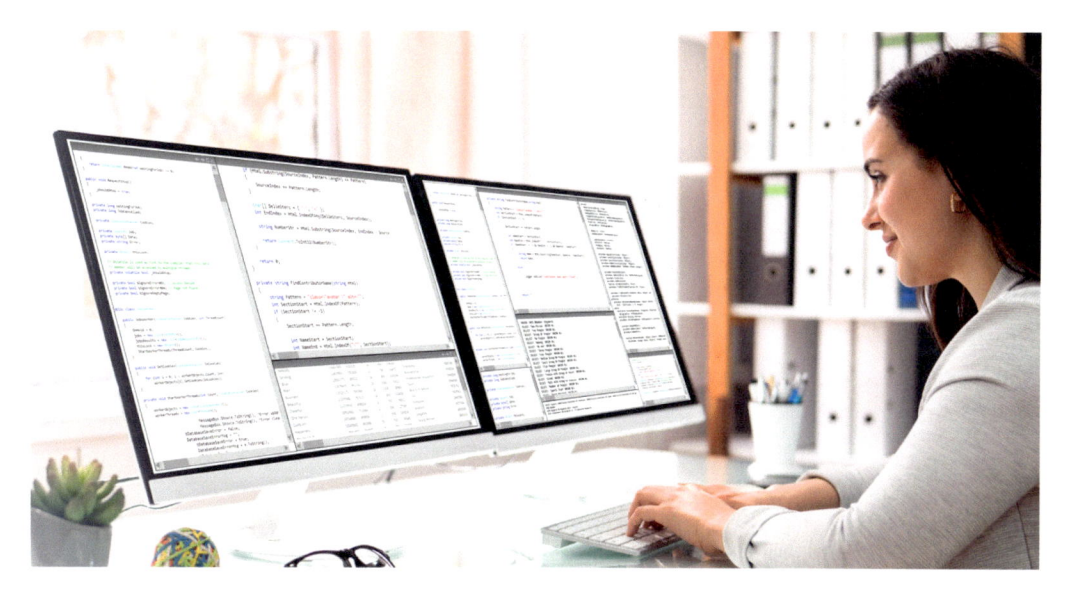

This increased screen time has been associated with a number of vision and general health issues, including digital eye strain, light sensitivity, dry eye, headaches, sleep disruption, and possibly mental health issues.

To counteract the potential adverse effects of blue light and screen time on our eyes and overall health, the macular carotenoids - lutein and zeaxanthin - have been shown to be effective.

For dry eye issues associated with tear evaporation from decreased blinking during long durations of screen time, supplementation with omega 3 and 6 fatty acids can also provide benefits.

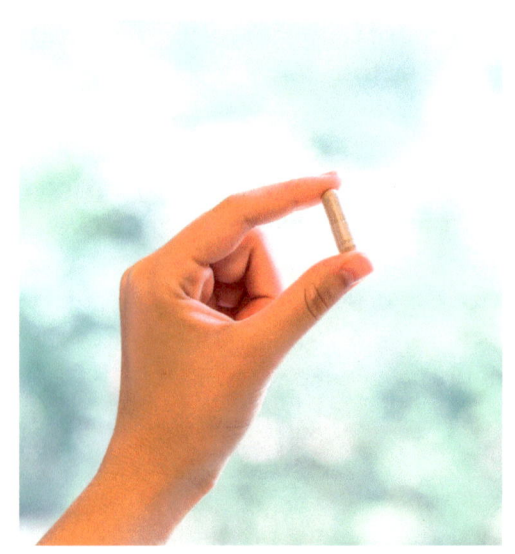

For all these reasons that we are facing leading to a lack of adequate nutritional support for our eyes from foods, it is my strong belief that *everyone* should take supplements for their vision.

This applies not only to older adults, the population believed to be the most at risk, but also to younger adults, teenagers, and children alike.

So, which specific supplements should you take to protect and preserve your precious eyes to ensure healthy vision for the years ahead? In the next section, I will share with you the perfect combination of dietary supplements that you should seek out for your precious eyesight.

Beyond Standard Supplements

As I shared in Parts I and II of this book, our eyes are complex organs with over 40 working parts. They need over 30 nutrients to keep them healthy.

Just as how you need to go *beyond* carrots and *beyond* beta carotene when it comes to the foods and nutrients important to support your eyes, similarly, you need to go *beyond* standard supplements for your eye health.

To best provide your eyes with the full spectrum of nutrients they need, I strongly believe it is necessary to take not just *one* supplement for your vision, but a *combination* of several supplements - 4 specific formulations, to be exact. You may already be taking three of these as part of your supplement routine. However, it is prudent to check the ingredients on the labels to ensure you are going *beyond* standard supplements to fully support your eyes.

In this next section, I will explain in more detail the 4 supplement types I believe are essential AND required for optimal eye health and prevention of eye disease-

- a multivitamin with bioflavonoids
- a macular carotenoid blend +
- a complete omega blend
- a diverse probiotic.

Beyond The Standard Multivitamin

According to surveys of adults in the U.S., approximately one-third of people take a multivitamin. This supplement typically contains-

- B vitamins involved in energy production by mitochondria - thiamine, riboflavin, niacin, biotin, pyridoxine, folate, and cobalamin (B12)
- vitamins A, C, and E for their roles as antioxidants to support eye and skin health and structural support
- vitamin D2 or D3 - beneficial for immune and hormone function
- minerals - calcium, iron, potassium, magnesium, zinc, and selenium as building blocks and cofactors in enzymatic reactions
- vitamin K - for healthy blood clotting

Though these types of multivitamins provide many nutrients, when it comes to your eye health, they may not provide you with ALL the nutritional support your eyes need. What are most of these standard multivitamins missing? Bioflavonoids!

Bioflavonoids

Phytonutrients called bioflavonoids are important to fully support your vision. As I described in Part I, bioflavonoids are a group of plant-derived compounds that help protect plants from oxidative stress, infection, and inflammation.

When obtained either through diet or as in supplement form, these bioflavonoids act similarly within the human body as antioxidants, anti-microbial compounds, and anti-inflammatory nutrients. Bioflavonoids can confer protection against disease caused by oxidative stress, infection, and inflammation.

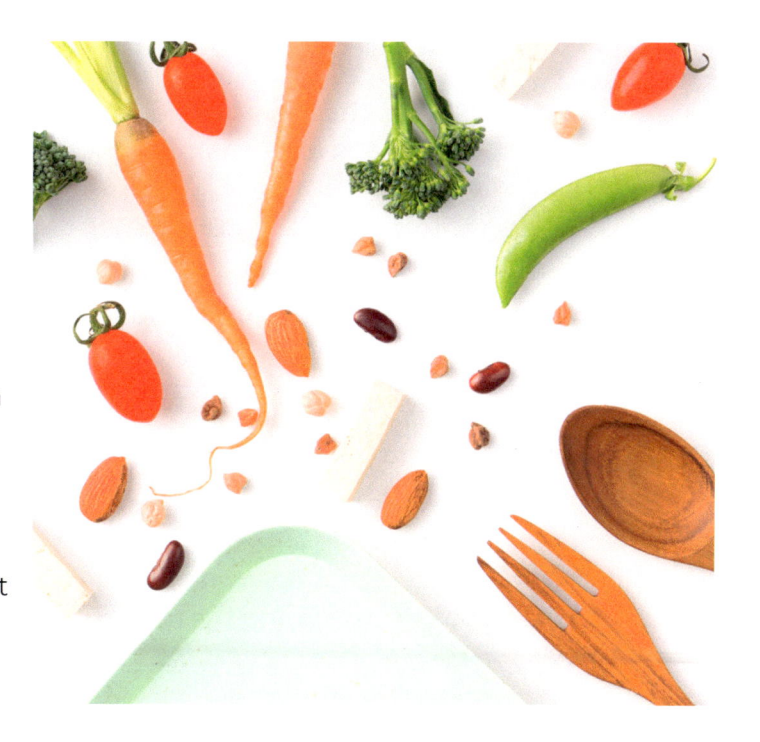

Research has shown that bioflavonoids like quercetin, resveratrol, sulforaphane glucosinolates, rutin, hesperidin, apigenin, naringenin, and allicin, amongst many others, are beneficial for retinal and optic nerve health.

The most commonly studied bioflavonoids for their eye health benefits include:

- Quercetin: This bioflavonoid is a potent antioxidant, also with anti-inflammatory properties. Studies have shown that quercetin may help protect the eyes from oxidative stress and reduce the risk of developing macular degeneration.

- Resveratrol: Found in red wine, red grapes, cherries, and apples, resveratrol has been shown to reduce vascular inflammation, improve blood vessel relaxation, and inhibit new blood vessel growth. Due to these vascular benefits, resveratrol is believed to support the eye's microcirculation, thereby helping prevent ocular diseases such as age-related macular degeneration, diabetic retinopathy, and glaucoma. Resveratrol has a high polyphenolic content and has also been shown to benefit cardiovascular health.

- Sulforaphane glucosinolates: Found in high concentrations in broccoli seeds and broccoli sprouts, this class of bioflavonoids has been shown in cell culture models to protect retinal pigment epithelial cells from oxidative stress and promote regeneration.

- Rutin and Hesperidin: These bioflavonoids are found in high concentrations in citrus fruits and have antioxidant and anti-inflammatory properties. Research has shown that both rutin and hesperidin may help improve blood flow to the eyes, reduce oxidative stress, and reduce the risk of developing macular degeneration.

- Anthocyanins: These bioflavonoids are a group of dark blue, purple, or red pigmented antioxidants found in dark fruits or vegetables such as blueberries, bilberries, aronia berries, dark blue grapes, acai fruit, cranberries, black raspberry, cherries, black currants, eggplant, and red cabbage. In the eye, anthocyanins such as blueberry and bilberry extracts have been shown to help fight oxidative stress in the retina, reduce inflammation, and provide anti-allergic, anti-microbial, anti-viral, and anti-cancer functions. Anthocyanins are also believed to support blood circulation and the health of small capillaries in the eye.

Thus, instead of taking just a standard multivitamin, you should seek out a formulation that provides a robust bioflavonoid blend to further support your retina, optic nerve, and cornea.

Unfortunately, most multivitamins are missing this important class of diverse plant-derived powerful nutrients. To fill in this important gap, I have formulated a multivitamin blend, with the inclusion of these key bioflavonoids customized for healthy vision.

My multivitamin with bioflavonoid product is called *Nourish*, and it is the foundational product in my supplement line, *Ageless by Dr. Rani*. Based on the available published research. this formulation provides the best combination of bioflavonoids to support eye health.

Nourish contains not only the bioflavonoids you need to maintain healthy vision - quercetin, citrus bioflavonoids, resveratrol, anthocyanins, broccoli blend, grape extract, and berry complex - but also the important vitamins and minerals, and antioxidants required for vision and overall health in their most bioavailable forms, including:

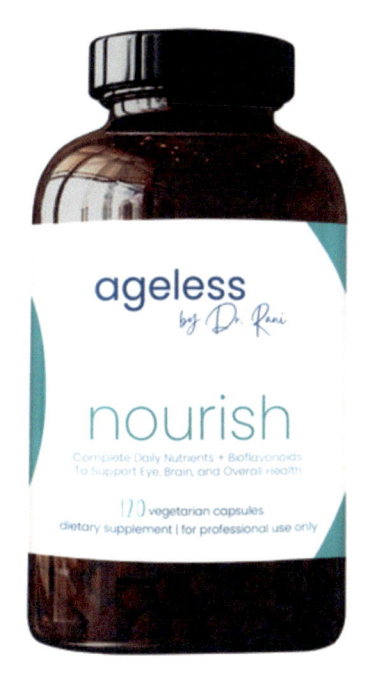

- Vitamins A: a mix of preformed vitamin A and provitamin A
- Vitamin C: two forms, as ascorbic acid and acerola
- Vitamin B1: two forms, as thiamine and benfotiamine
- Vitamins B2 & B6: phosphorylated forms: riboflavin-5'-phosphate and pyridoxal-5-phosphate, respectively
- Vitamin B3: two forms, as niacin and niacinamide
- Vitamin B5: two forms, as pantothenic acid and pantethine
- Vitamin B12: naturally occurring methylcobalamin form.
- Vitamin E Isomers: as tocotrienols from a high delta-tocotrienol annatto extract. Tocotrienols have higher antioxidant activity and unique benefits not observed with tocopherols.
- Vitamin D: intended to be augmented by endogenously synthesized vitamin D from sun exposure
- Vitamin K: provided as two naturally occurring forms—K1 and K2 to support bone metabolism and arterial health.

If you would like to learn more about *Nourish* and *Ageless by Dr. Rani*, my complete supplement line for eye and brain health, simply scan this QR code, or please visit my website, https://shop.rudranibanikmd.com/

Beyond the AREDS Supplements

The retina, the delicate 9-layered light-sensing tissue in the back of your eye, is quite vulnerable to oxidative stress. There is especially a concern for phototoxicity to the retina from exposure to high-energy ultraviolet (UV) rays and blue light wavelengths.

The macular carotenoids, lutein and zeaxanthin, are potent antioxidants. They are found in high concentrations in the macula, which is located at the center of the retina. Lutein and zeaxanthin help protect the macula from damage caused by oxidative stress and light exposure. These pigmented carotenoids function as your eyes' natural sunglasses and blue blockers.

Protecting Against Macular Degeneration

In age-related macular degeneration (AMD), a leading cause of blindness in the world, central vision can be lost due to damage to the macula. The root causes of AMD include oxidative stress, mitochondrial dysfunction, and inflammation.

Because of oxidative stress and mitochondrial dysfunction, waste deposits called "drusen" develop underneath the retina. As these drusen increase in number and size, inflammation then develops, which can lead to irreversible loss of function, retinal atrophy, new abnormal blood vessel growth, bleeding, and scarring.

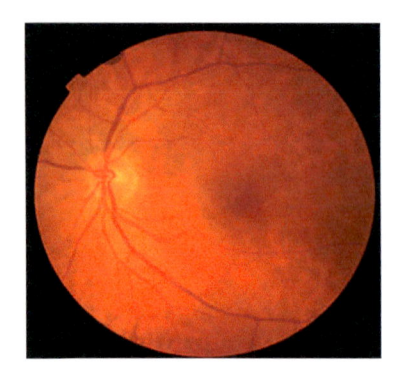

Normal macula 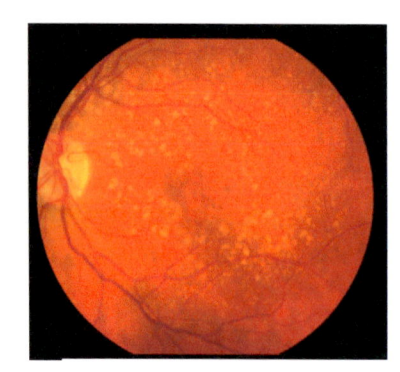 | Intermediate-stage dry AMD with drusen 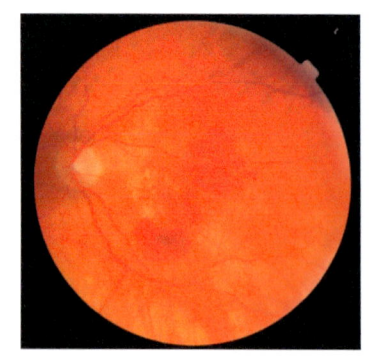 | Advanced wet AMD with bleeding

Numerous studies have shown that increased dietary intake of lutein and zeaxanthin may reduce the risk of developing macular degeneration. Higher levels of serum lutein are also associated with decreased risk of progression to advanced forms of macular degeneration.

The Age-Related Eye Disease Studies (AREDS) were two large clinical trials conducted by the National Eye Institute (NEI) to determine the effects of nutritional supplements on the progression of AMD.

The first trial, AREDS1, found that taking high doses of antioxidants (vitamins C and E), zinc, and copper can help slow down the progression of intermediate-stage AMD to advanced-stage AMD. This AREDS supplement contained the following ingredients:

- Vitamin C (500 mg)
- Vitamin E (400 IU)
- Beta-carotene (15 mg)
- Zinc (80 mg)
- Copper (2 mg)

AREDS1 found that this combination of vitamins and minerals reduced the risk of advanced AMD by 25% and the risk of vision loss by 19% in patients with intermediate or advanced AMD.

The second study, known as AREDS2, tested whether adding lutein and zeaxanthin or omega-3 fatty acids to the original AREDS formula would further reduce the risk of AMD progression. The study found that adding lutein and zeaxanthin to the formula was most beneficial in patients with baseline low levels of macular carotenoids. Adding omega-3 fatty acids (DHA 350 mg and EPA 650 mg) did not have a significant effect.

Based on both the AREDS1 and AREDS2 studies, the current AREDS supplement formulation* includes the following ingredients:

- Lutein (10 mg)
- Zeaxanthin (2mg)
- Vitamin C (500mg)
- Vitamin E (400IU)
- Zinc (80mg or 25mg)
- Copper (2 mg)

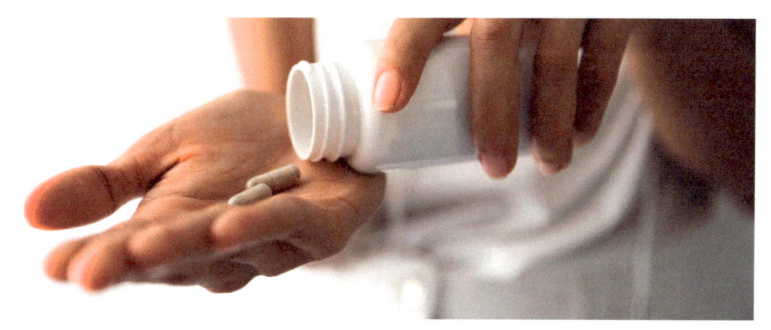

*Note that in this formulation, lutein and zeaxanthin replace beta-carotene, which has been associated with an increased risk of lung cancer in smokers.

It is important to keep in mind that this specific AREDS2 formulation is recommended only for patients with intermediate-stage AMD to prevent progression to an advanced stage with vision loss. There is no supplement that has been studied prospectively on a large scale for patients with early AMD or advanced AMD. There is also no study to date using supplements for the prevention of AMD for those who may not yet be diagnosed, but have risk factors, such as positive family history, history of smoking, presence of AMD genetic markers, etc.

Though the AREDS studies were landmark studies and have been instrumental in guiding the management of intermediate AMD, they had several major drawbacks.

First, the formulations included limited ingredients and conferred only a 25% reduction in risk, for only the subgroup of patients with intermediate AMD. Why did more people **not** benefit? As I have shared in previous chapters, there are many more nutrients that can help protect the retina by fighting the root causes of vision loss in AMD - oxidative stress, mitochondrial dysfunction, and inflammation. I believe that the lack of full nutritional support for the retina by the AREDS formulations led to suboptimal outcomes.

Since the AREDS1 and AREDS2 studies were published in 2001 and 2013, respectively, additional important nutrients for macular health have come into the spotlight. These nutrients were not included in the original formulations studied. However, these nutrients may be even more powerful in the fight against AMD and include:

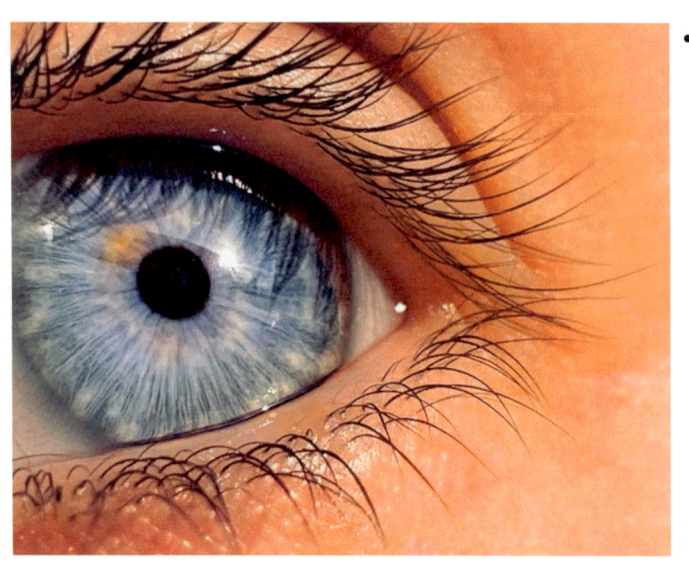

- Meso-zeaxanthin: A chemical cousin to zeaxanthin, meso-zeaxanthin is perhaps the most important and powerful of the macular carotenoids. It is concentrated at the very center of the macula, in the foveola. As an antioxidant, meso-zeaxanthin protects the part of the retina that allows us to see high-resolution 20/20 vision. An ingredient known as Lutemax® 2020 contains all three of the macular carotenoids (20 mg of lutein and 4 mg of a zeaxanthin/meso-zeaxanthin blend), and can provide full protection to the macula.

- Astaxanthin: A cousin to the macular carotenoids that are yellow pigments, astaxanthin is red in color. It is produced by a resilient species of algae (Haematococcus pluvialis), and can also be found in the marine species that consume these algae. Astaxanthin is the most potent of all known antioxidants. In one study, astaxanthin was found to be more powerful than alpha-tocopherol (a form of vitamin E), lycopene, beta-carotene (a precursor to vitamin A), lutein, and alpha-carotene.

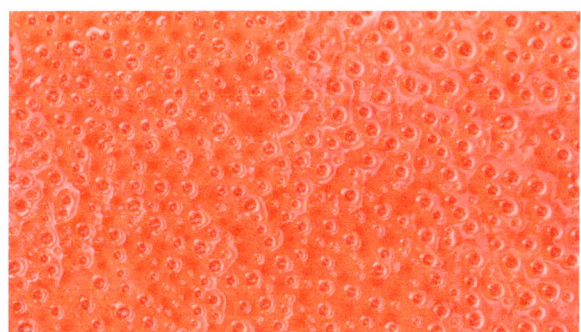

  The red color of this algae comes from the powerful antioxidant carotenoid, astaxanthin.

  Astaxanthin, in conjunction with the macular carotenoids, has been shown to benefit macular degeneration. It also has been shown to decrease free radicals after cataract surgery and improve blood flow in the choroid in the back of the eye. Research has also shown astaxanthin to offer many other health benefits, such as support of the immune system, cognitive health, skin, cardiovascular health, and fertility.

- Anthocyanins: As noted in the section above, deeply pigmented bioflavonoids are known as anthocyanins. Anthocyanins such as blueberry and bilberry extracts have been shown to help fight oxidative stress in the retina and reduce inflammation in cell culture models. Anthocyanins are also believed to support blood circulation and the health of small capillaries in the eye and thus may be beneficial for both macular degeneration as well as other retinal vascular disorders, such as diabetic retinopathy.

- Tocotrienol: Tocotrienol is a form of vitamin E that has a higher antioxidant activity and unique benefits not seen with the more common vitamin E isomers, namely the tocopherols. Vitamin E is important for the structural support of lipids found in cell membranes. It is especially important for the structural support of retinal cells because they have a high cell membrane turnover. Tocotrienols have been shown to inhibit oxidative damage to lipids in cell membranes. The delta-tocotrienol form has the greatest antioxidant properties among the tocotrienol isomers, and 3 to 5 times higher than the tocopherol forms of vitamin E.

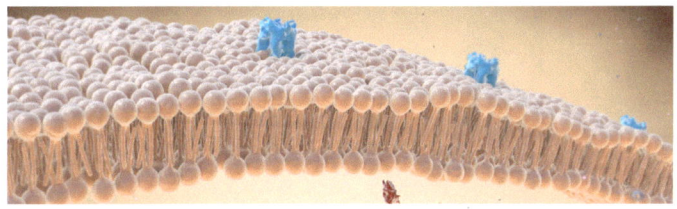

Tocotrienol plays a protective role as an antioxidant in maintaining the structural integrity of the cell membrane.

Aside from not including some of the very powerful antioxidant nutrients noted above, another drawback of the AREDS formulations is the high levels of zinc used. In the United States, the Recommended Dietary Allowance (RDA) of zinc for men is 11 mg per day, and for women is 8 mg per day. Levels above 40 mg per day may be harmful.

The original AREDS formulation used 80 mg per day. In addition, patients in the AREDS study were taking a daily multivitamin that provided another 11 mg, a cumulative dose that is well above the safety limits for daily zinc intake.

Some argue that very high zinc intake may confer health benefits and decrease mortality. However, on the flip side, such high zinc levels may negatively impact AMD. For example, a study from 2018 showed that individuals with certain genetic risk profiles for AMD (namely, high CFH and low ARMS2 profiles) are sensitive to high levels of zinc intake. With high zinc intake, these individuals developed worse outcomes and a two times higher risk for the progression of AMD. Though not yet widely performed, genetic testing for AMD genetic variants may help personalize nutritional and supplement recommendations for patients at risk for AMD.

Given these limitations of the AREDS studies, in order to fully protect your retina against AMD, when choosing eye health supplements, I strongly believe that you need to go *beyond* the AREDS formulation with respect to the ingredients and their dosing.

In addition to protecting the macula from macular degeneration, protecting against blue light and its potential adverse health effects is also of utmost concern, for both the young and old.

We live in a digital world in which we depend on our screens for work, education, social connection, and entertainment. The average daily time spent on screens has skyrocketed to over 10 hours for adults and 6 hours for children.

Though our devices have become indispensable, they can put a significant strain on our eyes. Excessive blue light exposure from screens has been associated with digital eye strain, as well as sleep disruption, mental health issues, and even attention disorders (notably in children).

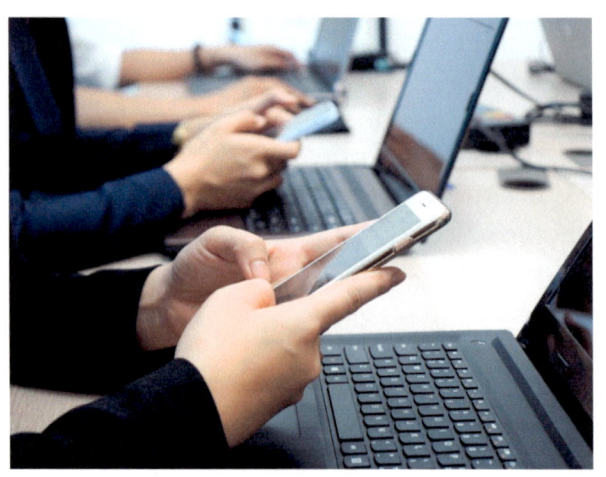

Fortunately, macular carotenoids have been shown to reduce many symptoms of eye strain associated with screen use. In the B.L.U.E. study, 48 adults with high screen time exposure took a supplement with Lutemax® 2020 for 6 months. They had significant improvement in their macular pigment ocular density (MPOD, an objective measure of the concentrations of the macular carotenoids in the retina), as well as their visual performance measures, sleep quality, eye strain, visual fatigue, and frequent headaches compared to a placebo. Another study of adults with at least 4 hours of daily screen time improved contrast sensitivity, sleep quality, reduced eye fatigue, eyestrain, and headaches with a macular carotenoid supplement compared to a placebo.

If you are interested in protecting your eyes from macular degeneration, a leading cause of preventable blindness, as well as from the potential adverse vision and general health effects of excessive blue light exposure from screens, I urge you to be proactive.

First and foremost, be sure that you are getting the full range of nutrients your eyes need from your diet to support your eye health. Also, make eye-healthy lifestyle choices, such as using UV protection in the form of sunglasses or a wide-brimmed hat when outdoors, stopping smoking, exercising regularly, maintaining a healthy weight, and limiting screen time before bed. These strategies are the foundation for healthy vision.

In addition, to give your eyes the full protection they need, I urge you to consider taking an eye health supplement. Choose a formulation specifically formulated with the science-backed ingredients I described above, such as:

- all three of the macular carotenoids - lutein, zeaxanthin, and meso-zeaxanthin (preferably in the form of Lutemax® 2020)
- astaxanthin
- anthocyanins (preferably from a berry blend extract)
- delta-tocotrienol
- low to no zinc (if you are already including adequate sources of zinc in your diet and are taking a multivitamin containing zinc)

Also, keep in mind that this formulation designed to fortify your retinal health should be *in addition* to a complete multivitamin with the full range of bioflavonoids that support eye health, as noted in the section above.

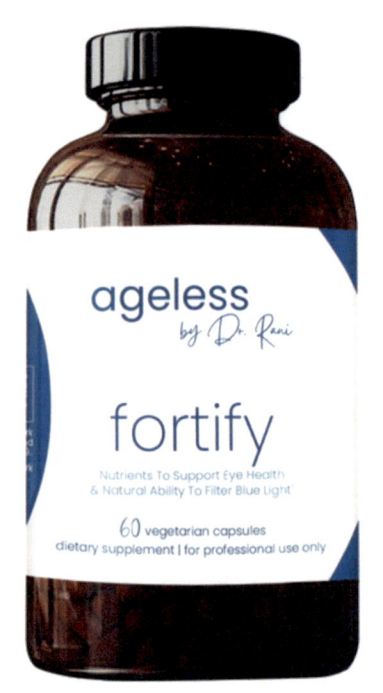

Unfortunately, most vitamins on the market for AMD or blue light protection are missing one or more of these important powerful nutrients. To fill in this important gap, I have formulated a macular carotenoid blend, with the inclusion of additional botanicals for vision health.

My macular carotenoid + product is called *Fortify*, and it is the flagship product in my supplement line, *Ageless by Dr. Rani.* Based on the available published research, I designed this formulation to provide the best combination of carotenoids PLUS botanicals to support your retina, optic nerve, and lens - lutein, zeaxanthin, meso-zeaxanthin, astaxanthin, anthocyanins, delta-tocotrienol, and ginkgo biloba.

If you would like to learn more about *Fortify* and *Ageless by Dr. Rani,* my complete supplement line for eye and brain health, simply scan this QR code, or please visit my website, https://shop.rudranibanikmd.com/

Beyond Standard Omega-3s

The Omegas

Omega fatty acids are well known to play roles in maintaining vision, brain, and overall health. This fatty acid nutrient class includes the omega-3s and omega-6s and the lesser-known omega-7s and omega-9s.

The two key omega-3 fatty acids, EPA and DHA, are essential and serve as building blocks for cell membranes. In fact, the highest concentration of DHA in the body is found in the retinal photoreceptors as part of the outer segments of their cell membranes. Because the outer segments process light energy and have a high turnover rate, a constant supply of DHA is crucial for optimum retinal health.

The omega-3s also serve as antioxidants and anti-inflammatory nutrients. They have been shown to reduce oxidative stress, which may in turn reduce the risk for diseases such as stroke, heart disease, eczema, and other autoimmune conditions like lupus and rheumatoid arthritis.

A high dietary intake of omega-3 fatty acids has been proven to be helpful for ocular conditions such as dry eye. Studies have also shown that a diet high in omega-3 fatty acids may improve visual acuity and reduce the risk of developing macular degeneration. In animal models, omega-3 fatty acids have been shown to reduce inflammatory mediators in uveitis, which is inflammation inside the eye.

Omega-6 fatty acids can have dual effects on eye health. On one hand, omega-6 fatty acids are essential for the body, important for structural support and maintaining healthy cell membranes. However, excess intake of omega-6 fatty acids is converted into arachidonic acid, leading the body down the inflammatory pathways. With respect to vision health, high omega-6 dietary intake has been associated with a higher risk for advanced forms of macular degeneration.

When it comes to omega-6 and omega-3, though both are essential nutrients, the ratio between intake of the two is most critical. The suggested omega 6:3 ratio for promoting health and limiting inflammation is 4:1.

Unfortunately, people on the Western "Standard American Diet" (S.A.D.) who consume high amounts of omega-6 fatty acids, ultra-processed food, and high levels of simple sugars tend to have omega 6:3 ratios that are much higher, some in the range of 12:1, 30:1, or even 50:1!

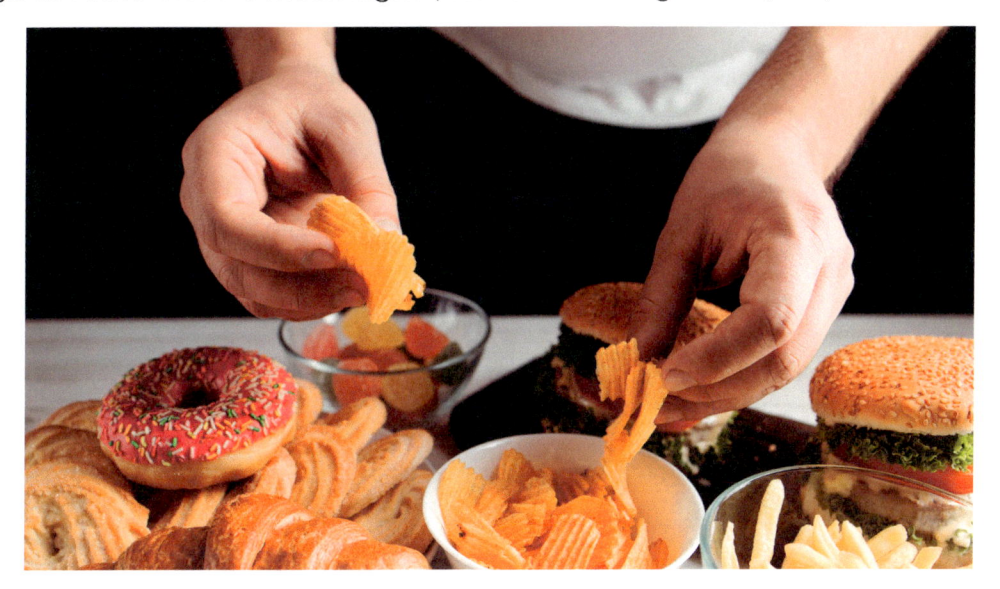

Ultra-processed, fried, and packaged baked foods tend to contain high levels of omega-6 fatty acids, that can promote inflammatory pathways within the body.

It is important to note that not all omega-6 fatty acids are pro-inflammatory. One particular omega-6 fatty acid known as gamma-linolenic acid (GLA), is converted by the body into dihomo-gamma-linolenic acid (DGLA), which is anti-inflammatory.

GLA can be found in plant-based oils, such as evening primrose oil, borage oil, and black currant seed oil.

When given in conjunction with the omega-3 fatty acids, DHA and EPA, GLA has been shown in clinical studies to benefit dry eye and improve ocular inflammatory markers.

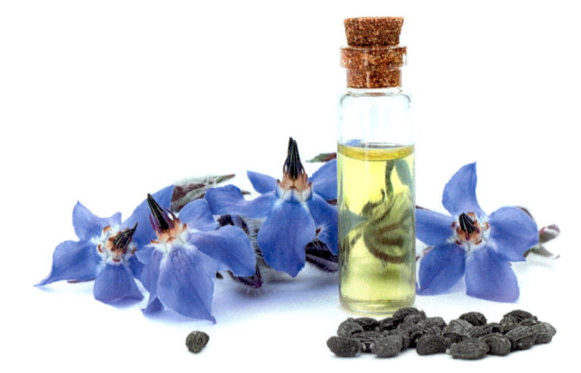

Borage oil, an excellent source of the anti-inflammatory omega-6, gamma-linolenic acid (GLA)

Omega-7 fatty acids, such as palmitoleic acid, are found in relatively low levels in most diets. However, there is emerging evidence that omega-7 fatty acids may have potent anti-inflammatory and antioxidant effects, which could be especially beneficial for eye health.

Several studies have been published investigating the potential benefits of omega-7s in treating dry eye syndrome. One study involved patients with dry eye syndrome who were given a supplement containing omega-7s with other nutrients for three months. The results showed a significant improvement in symptoms and signs of dry eye compared to the placebo group. Another study using sea buckthorn oil, an excellent source of omega-7 fatty acids, showed improved tear film osmolarity, a marker for dry eye syndrome.

Finally, omega-9 fatty acids, such as oleic acid, are found in high amounts in olive, macadamia nut, and other vegetable oils. Strong evidence suggests that a Mediterranean-style diet high in monounsaturated fatty acids (including the omega-9s) is associated with a reduced risk of age-related macular degeneration.

Overall, there is strong evidence for the eye health benefits of omega-3 fatty acids. There is also compelling emerging evidence to support the potential benefits of omega-6 (gamma-linolenic acid, GLA), omega-7 (palmitoleic acid), and omega-9 (oleic acid) fatty acids for eye health.

Maintaining a healthy and balanced diet that includes various fats to support your eye health is of utmost importance and should be the foundation for nutritional support for vision. However, to fully support your eye and overall health, I believe that we all need to go beyond diet and fill in any nutrient gaps.

As I shared in the sections above, when seeking out supplements for eye health, it is prudent to go beyond standard multivitamins by choosing a multivitamin with bioflavonoids and to go beyond the standard AREDS formulations by choosing a macular carotenoid blend that also has additional antioxidant ingredients. Similarly, it is just as prudent to take a full-spectrum omega supplement *beyond* the standard omega-3.

Most omega supplements marketed for eye health only provide the better-known omega-3 fatty acids, DHA and EPA. A few formulations contain the omega-6 fatty acid, GLA, as well. Omega 7 and 9 are typically not included in most brands available. Fortunately, you can fill in the missing pieces of the omega puzzle by choosing a more robust and powerful omega formulation to protect your vision for the years and decades to come.

To fill in this omega gap, I have formulated an omega blend that includes highly absorbable omega 3 (DHA and EPA from fish oil), omega-6 (GLA from borage oil), omega-7 (palmitoleic acid from virgin organic macadamia nut oil), and omega-9 (oleic acid from a combination of virgin organic macadamia nut oil and borage oil).

Based on the available research and my extensive experience managing patients for over twenty years, I believe this curated combination of omegas affords the best, most complete omega support. This blend has offered protection for my patients with inflammatory eye conditions such as severe dry eye, as well as early, intermediate, and advanced forms of macular degeneration,

My complete omega blend product is called *Soothe*, and it is a key product in my supplement line, *Ageless by Dr. Rani.*

To learn more about *Soothe* and *Ageless by Dr. Rani*, my complete supplement line for eye and brain health, simply scan this QR code or please visit my website, https://shop.rudranibanikmd.com/

Beyond the Standard Probiotic

As I shared in Part I, research suggests that there is a strong connection between the health of your gut microbiome and your overall health, including your eye health. A healthy gut microbiome is essential for maintaining a strong immune system, which can in turn help protect your eyes from infections and diseases.

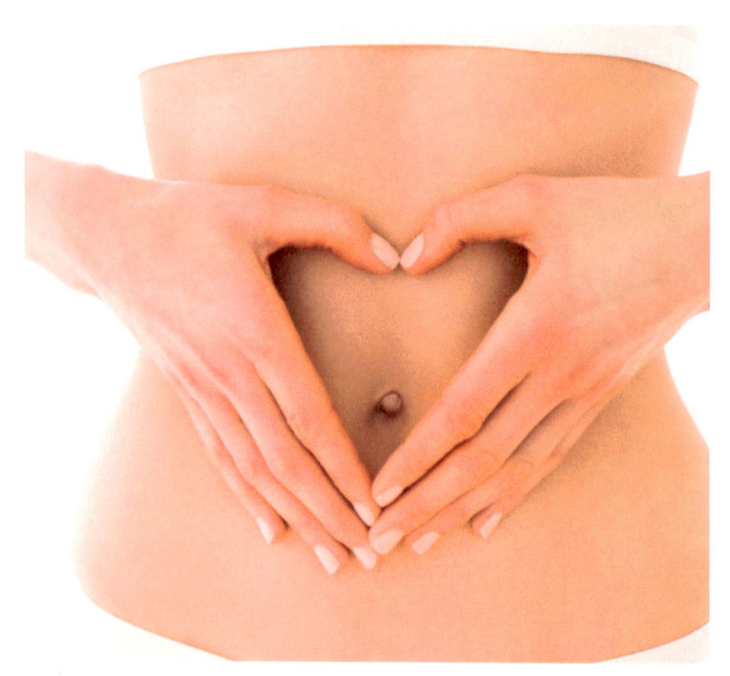

One way in which a healthy gut microbiome can benefit your eye health is by reducing inflammation. Chronic inflammation in the body has been linked to several eye diseases, including macular degeneration, dry eye, glaucoma, and uveitis. By reducing inflammation, a healthy gut microbiome can help reduce the risk of developing these diseases.

Another way in which a healthy gut microbiome can benefit your eye health is by producing essential nutrients. Gut bacteria can produce vitamins and other nutrients that are important for maintaining healthy eyes, such as vitamin A, which is essential for vision.

Probiotics, which are beneficial bacteria that are found in certain foods and supplements, can help support a healthy gut microbiome and potentially improve eye health. Studies have shown that probiotics can reduce inflammation and improve immune function, both of which are important for maintaining healthy eyes.

Additionally, gut dysbiosis, which is an imbalance of gut bacteria, has been linked to several ophthalmic diseases. For example, a study found that individuals with dry eye disease had a different composition of gut bacteria compared to healthy individuals. Several other studies have found that patients with uveitis and macular degeneration had altered gut microbiomes compared to healthy controls..

The research linking gut dysbiosis to eye disease is still in its infancy. Much more needs to be explored and understood with respect to the imbalance between pathogenic organisms ("bad bacteria") and commensal organisms ("good bacteria"), and their potential links to specific ocular conditions.

Nevertheless, striving for a healthy gut microbiome is important, not only for your eye health but for your general health. As I have mentioned time and time again in this book, diet is the foundation when it comes to supporting a healthy gut microbiome.

Adding live-culture foods to your diet, as found in probiotic-rich foods like yogurt, sauerkraut, kimchi, and kombucha, helps support your gut microbiome and potentially reduces the risk of developing ophthalmic diseases.

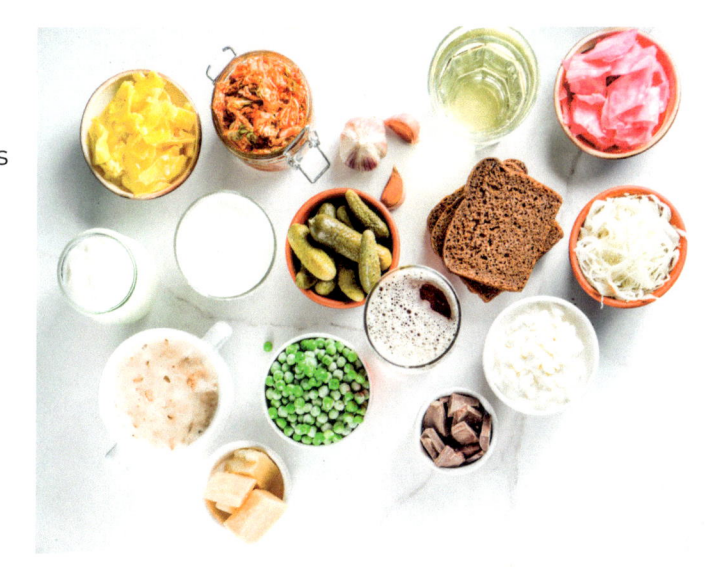

In addition to live probiotics in your diet, I've also found that taking a probiotic supplement can be highly beneficial. When choosing a probiotic supplement to help maintain healthy vision and proactively ward off eye diseases, it is important to look for these three features:

- diversity of bacterial strains
- a high count of live bacteria at the time of manufacture (colony forming units, or CFUs)
- shelf stability

While probiotic supplements can have potential health benefits, not all probiotic supplements are created equal. Generic or low-quality probiotic supplements may have several pitfalls, which could impact their effectiveness and safety.

Firstly, generic probiotic supplements may not disclose the specific strains or CFU counts of the probiotics used in their formulations. Without this information, it's difficult to know if the supplement contains strains that have been researched for their potential health benefits or if the CFU count is high enough to provide a therapeutic effect.

Secondly, generic supplements may not have undergone rigorous quality control or testing to ensure that the probiotics are viable, stable, and safe. This could result in lower potency or contamination, which could reduce the effectiveness or even cause harm.

Lastly, generic probiotic supplements may not be formulated to address specific health concerns or conditions, making them less effective for addressing those issues.

In contrast to possible issues with generic formulations, premium brands of probiotic supplements typically have higher standards for quality and transparency. Premium brand labels typically disclose the specific strains and CFU counts used in their formulations and undergo rigorous testing and quality control to ensure that their products are viable, stable, and safe. Additionally, premium brands may formulate their products to address specific health concerns or conditions, which could result in more targeted and effective results.

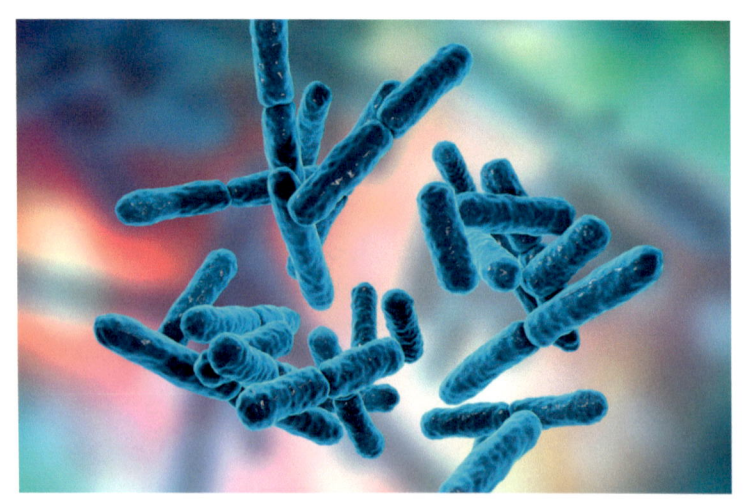

Overall, it's important to choose a premium brand of probiotic supplement to ensure that you are getting a high-quality product that is safe, effective, and formulated to address your specific health concerns. While these supplements may be more expensive than generic brands, the benefits they provide may be well worth the extra investment.

Based on my research in gut dysbiosis and ocular disease, I have curated a probiotic formulation that includes bacterial strains that I believe best promote eye health. My probiotic formulation, *Balance*, consists of 10 of the most highly-researched probiotic strains, each with a specific CFU count listed.

Its special formulation for eye health sets *Balance* apart from standard probiotics. For example, *Lactobacillus rhamnosus GG*, one of the key bacterial strains in *Balance,* has antimicrobial properties and may help boost the immune system to fend off bacterial infections. This particular probiotic strain has been studied for vernal conjunctivitis, a form of allergic eye inflammation.

Balance also offers select *Lactobacillus* and *Bifidobacterium* strains that have solid clinical research to back their benefits for multiple aspects of health. Incorporating a diverse probiotic supplement into your daily routine can thus support your eye, gastrointestinal, and overall health.

These strains are robust and capable of surviving the harsh journey to the intestines, where they can attach to the intestinal walls and function effectively to support gastrointestinal health.

The survivability of the strains is further assisted by delayed-release technology and unique moisture-resistant, desiccant-lined packaging. This means that *Balance* does not require refrigeration, making it convenient for travelers and anyone on the go.

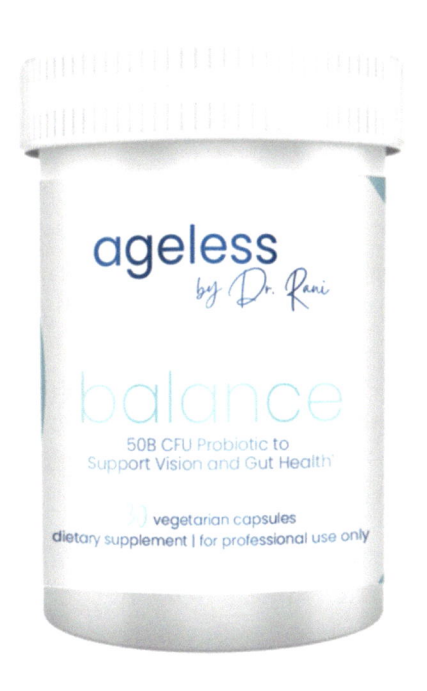

Instead of settling for an inexpensive standard probiotic supplement that may include only a handful of microbial strains that may have little to no research behind its efficacy or potency – be proactive and choose a highly potent, shelf-stable, dairy-free probiotic formulation specially formulated for eye health.

To learn more about *Balance* and *Ageless by Dr. Rani*, my complete supplement line for eye and brain health, simply scan this QR code or please visit my website, https://shop.rudranibanikmd.com/

In summary, when it comes to supplements to protect and preserve your vision, or possibly even help address chronic inflammatory eye conditions like dry eye or macular degeneration, I believe it is best to take a combination of formulations -

- a multivitamin with bioflavonoids
- a macular carotenoids blend + with astaxanthin, berry extract, and tocotrienol
- a complete omega blend (omegas 3, 6, 7, and 9) and
- a diverse probiotic with multiple strains, a high CFU count, and shelf stable.

If you are one of the millions of people who already take 3 out of these 4 types of formulations (a multivitamin, an omega, and a probiotic), to give your eyes extra protection, especially against the intense visual demands of today's digital world, I would suggest adding a macular carotenoid blend to your daily regimen.

Also, if you would like to learn more about any of the four supplement formulations that make up *Ageless by Dr. Rani,* my complete supplement line for eye and brain health, simply scan the QR codes below, or please visit my website, https://shop.rudranibanikmd.com/

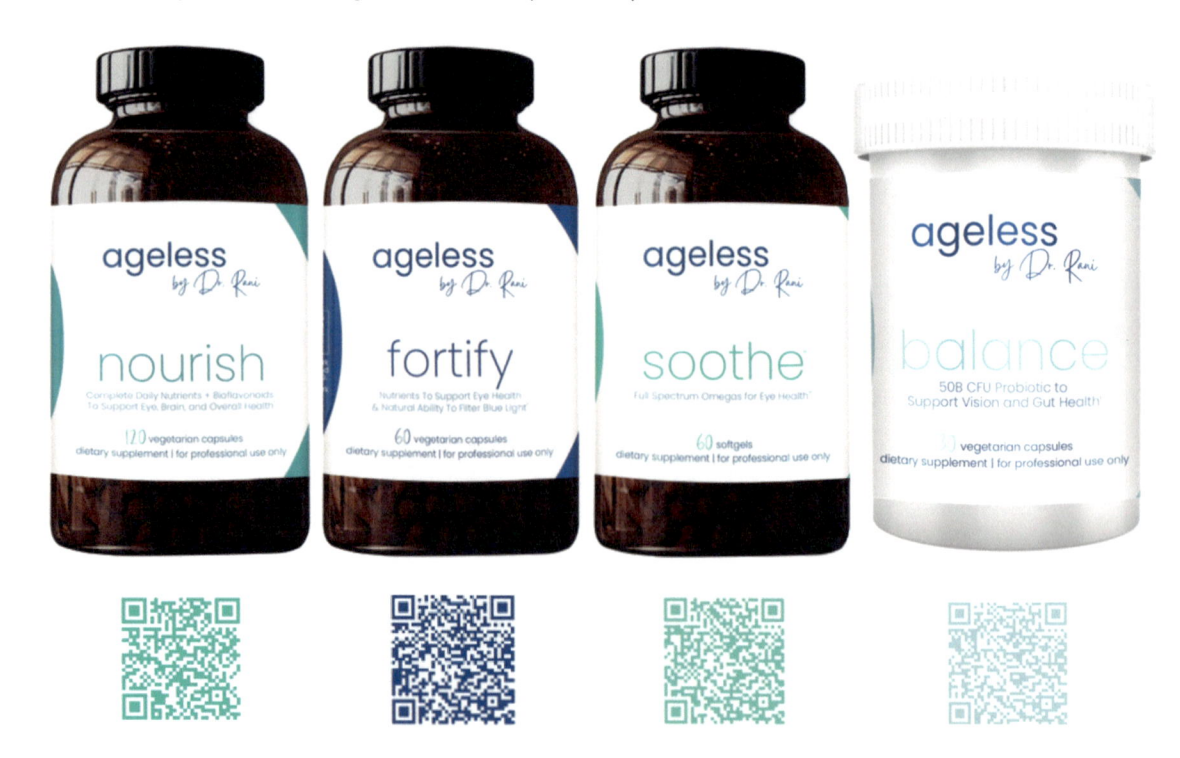

Additional Resources

Free Resources

If you'd like a deeper explanation of some of the topics I discuss in this book or would like to explore more foods that benefit your eyes, I offer several free eBooks -

- What are Integrative and Functional Medicine?
- Eye Anatomy 101 and
- Best Foods For Eye Health - A to Z Supplement.

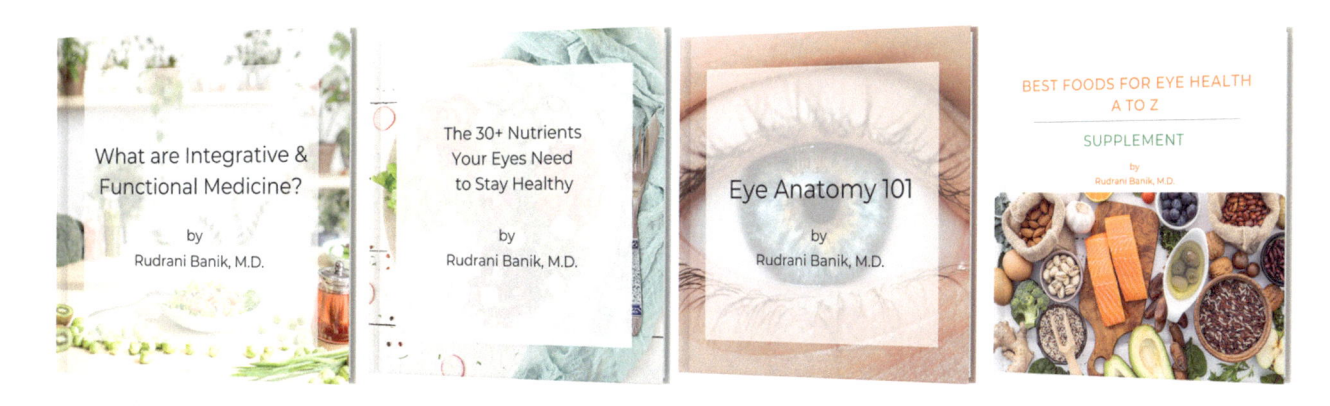

You may find these useful resources that are companions to 'Beyond Carrots' via my website, https://rudranibanikmd.com/beyondcarrots or scan the QR code below and click on the tile that says "Download Free Resources."

To unlock your FREE access, be sure to enter the secret word found in Part II of this book, which is the food that starts with the letter 'V."

Additional Resources

The Beyond Carrots Toolkit

To make healthy eye nutrition simpler for you, I have created several resources collectively called The Beyond Carrots Toolkit. This toolkit includes a collection of digital products designed to help you implement the nutritional strategies outlined in Parts I and II of this book.

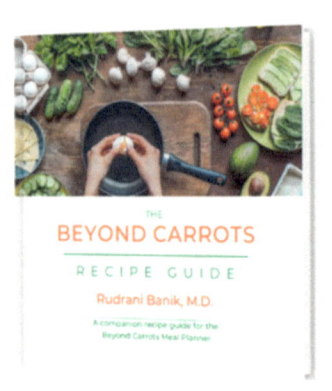

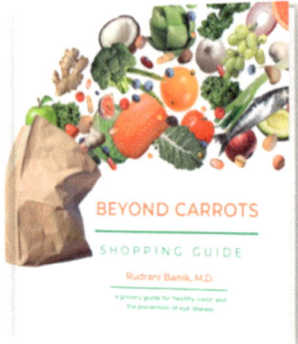

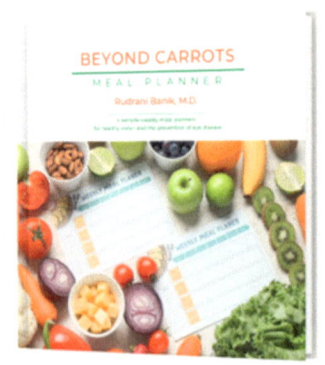

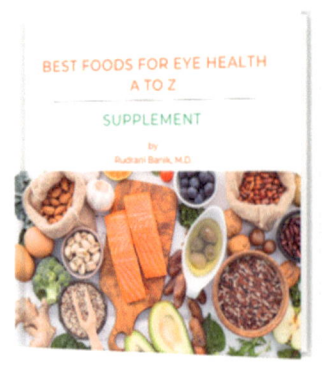

One resource in The Beyond Carrots Toolkit is "The Beyond Carrots Meal Planner." This 4-week sample meal planner incorporates eye-healthy, therapeutic foods mentioned in Part II of this book into a comprehensive food plan to provide complete nutrition for your eyes. There are vegetarian and vegan versions of the planner as well.

The toolkit also includes "The Beyond Carrots Recipe Guide" to pair with the food planner. This downloadable digital resource contains easy-to-make delicious, mouth-watering recipes for smoothies, salads, entrees, soups, beverages, and desserts that satisfy any palate.

In the toolkit, I have also compiled a grocery list of the best foods to promote your eye health called 'The Beyond Carrots Shopping Guide."

Finally, there are other eye-healthy foods that, due to space limitations, could not be included in this book. These supplemental foods, including select animal products packed with eye-healthy nutrients, are highlighted in the downloadable pdf, "Best Foods For Eye Health A to Z Supplement."

The Beyond Carrots Toolkit continued...

All of these additional resources-

- The Beyond Carrots Meal Planner
- The Beyond Carrots Recipe Guide
- The Beyond Carrots Shopping Guide and
- Best Foods For Eye Health A to Z Supplement

can be purchased by visiting my website, www.rudranibanikmd.com/toolkit or by scanning the QR code below with your smartphone camera.

The Beyond Carrots Cookbooks

if you enjoy fresh, homemade food that is not only healthy but will also support your eyes, you will absolutely love the *Beyond Carrots Cookbook*!

In this cookbook, I've curated over 200 delicious and nutritious recipes that will support healthy vision. The nutrients and foods found in the *Beyond Carrots Cookbook* will help keep your vision healthy and strong. They will also help ward off common eye diseases such as dry eye, cataracts, macular degeneration, and glaucoma.

The full-color illustrations will no doubt have your mouth watering. This cookbook will be a feast for your eyes and your palate!

To serve all styles of eating, I also offer vegetarian and vegan versions of the cookbook. The entire series is available on Amazon and on Kindle as well. Just scan the QR codes under your book of choice to order your print or digital copy today!

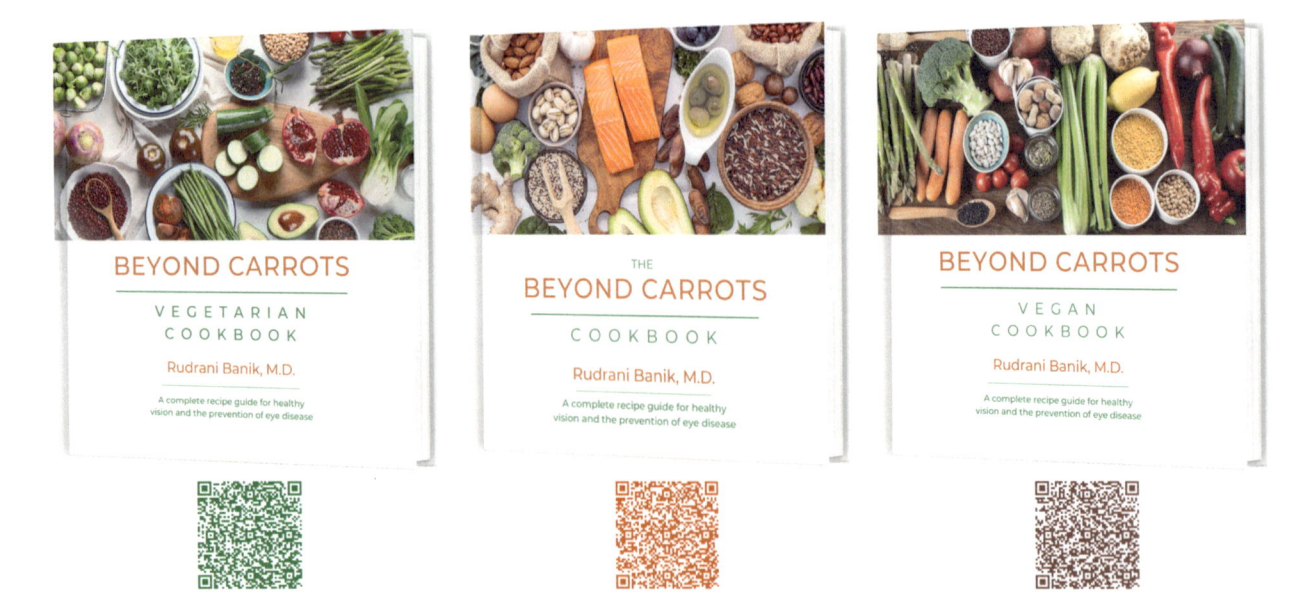

P.S. - The *Beyond Carrots Cookbooks* also make great gifts, so be sure to share them with your family and friends. They will be forever grateful to you not only for introducing them to a healthier way of eating but also for helping them preserve the precious gift of vision!

The Nutrition Eye-Q Test

Also, if you haven't already, please take the **Nutrition Eye-Q Test** on my website. This quick online assessment is a tool that will guide you toward personalized eye-healthy nutrients and foods you need to keep your vision strong.

By answering simple questions about your medical and eye history, current diet, and lifestyle habits, you will receive a personalized report. This individualized report will highlight which nutrients and foods you should focus on based on the 4 categories described at the end of Part I:

- C - Cornea, Conjunctiva, and Tear Film
- L - Lens
- O - Optic Nerve and Trabecular Meshwork
- R - Retina

Your **Nutrition Eye-Q** results (C, L, O, R) will serve as your guide to the foods highlighted in Part II of this book, so you can keep your eyes healthy and eat right for your sight!

To take the free online **Nutrition Eye-Q Test**, simply scan this QR code with your smartphone camera:

Be sure to tell your family and friends about the **Nutrition Eye-Q Test** assessment so they too may benefit from a personalized eye nutrition plan.

I hope that you will find all these additional resources indispensable and that with their help, you will enjoy excellent vision for years and decades to come.

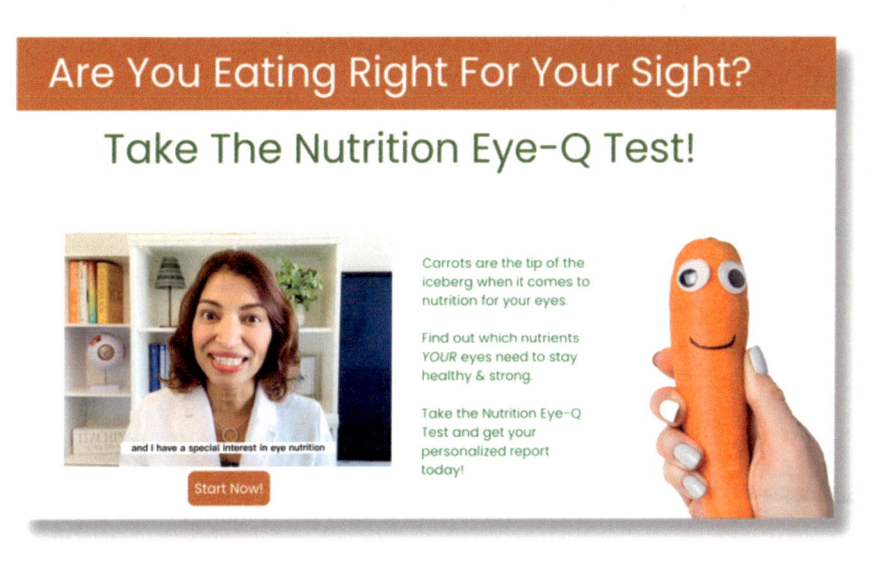

Acknowledgments

This book would not have been possible without the collective work of many who have come before me, those who have dedicated their lives to understanding vision and nutrition. From the traditional Western medicine perspective, I owe a debt of gratitude to the researchers in ocular physiology and pathophysiology who worked tirelessly to better our understanding of disease processes that affect the eye.

I want to thank the educators and community of the Institute for Functional Medicine (IFM), who are firm believers in the power of food as medicine. I am also grateful for the Mindshare and Mastermind communities, a group of forward-thinking practitioners who are always available for support and love. I am incredibly thankful for my amazing colleagues in the nutritional space. Special thanks to Ashley Koff, RD, Dr. Kellyann Petrucci, and JJ Virgin for their endless support.

I owe a debt of gratitude to my entire team, who helped me behind the scenes, with a special thank you to Sophia Forbes, who helped me in the primary research for the best foods for eye health A to Z.

I also owe tremendous gratitude to one of my dearest friends, Kristin Mathis. Without her editing genius and endearing support, I would not have been able to refine this manuscript.

And of course, there is my family - my husband, Sandeep, and daughter, Lylah- thank you for enduring the ups and downs during my writing journey, being sounding boards for ideas, and for your endless love and support. A special thank you to Lylah, who has an eye for aesthetics well beyond her 14 years and was instrumental in creating this book's beautiful design and layout.

And last but not least, I need to thank my patients. I may have learned the science of medicine and ophthalmology through years of schooling. Still, you all taught me something much more valuable than anything I could have ever learned from a textbook or classroom - the art of being a physician—a sincere debt of gratitude.

References

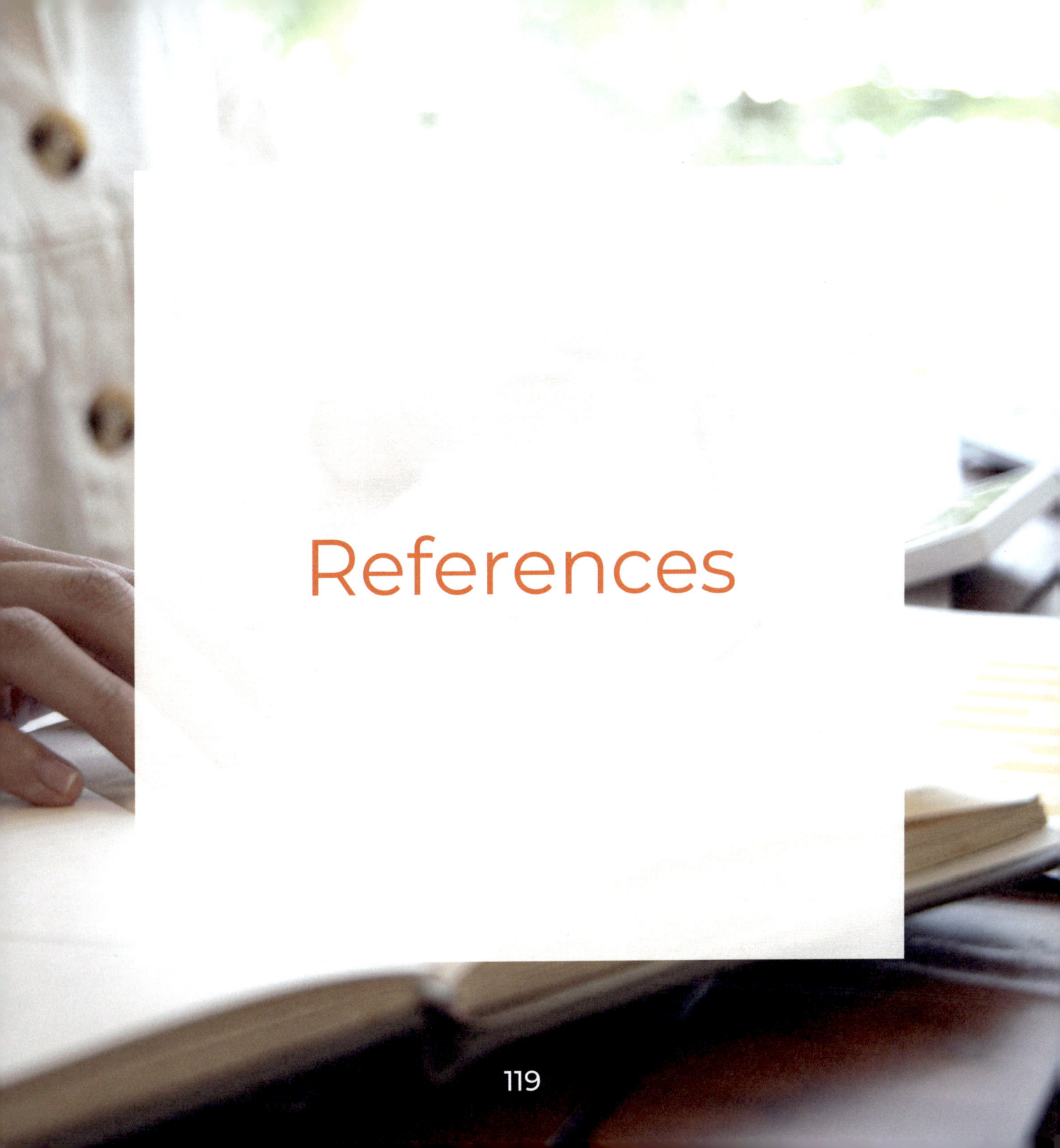

1. Abdel-Aal el-SM, Akhtar H, Zaheer K, Ali R. Dietary sources of lutein and zeaxanthin carotenoids and their role in eye health. Nutrients. 2013 Apr 9;5(4):1169-85. doi: 10.3390/nu5041169. PMID: 23571649; PMCID: PMC3705341.

2. Abidi W, Jiménez S, Moreno MÁ, Gogorcena Y. Evaluation of antioxidant compounds and total sugar content in a nectarine [Prunus persica (L.) Batsch] progeny. Int J Mol Sci. 2011;12(10):6919-35. doi: 10.3390/ijms12106919. Epub 2011 Oct 19. PMID: 22072927; PMCID: PMC3211018.

3. Abu-Amero KK, Kondkar AA, Chalam KV. Resveratrol and Ophthalmic Diseases. Nutrients. 2016 Apr 5;8(4):200. doi: 10.3390/nu8040200. PMID: 27058553; PMCID: PMC4848669.

4. Adachi S, Sawada N, Yuki K, Uchino M, Iwasaki M, Tsubota K, Tsugane S. Intake of Vegetables and Fruits and the Risk of Cataract Incidence in a Japanese Population: The Japan Public Health Center-Based Prospective Study. J Epidemiol. 2021 Jan 5;31(1):21-29. doi: 10.2188/jea.JE20190116. Epub 2019 Dec 14. PMID: 31839643; PMCID: PMC7738640.

5. Adomėnienė A, Venskutonis PR. Dioscorea spp.: Comprehensive Review of Antioxidant Properties and Their Relation to Phytochemicals and Health Benefits. Molecules. 2022 Apr 17;27(8):2530. doi: 10.3390/molecules27082530. PMID: 35458730; PMCID: PMC9026138.

6. Age-Related Eye Disease Study 2 Research Group. Lutein + zeaxanthin and omega-3 fatty acids for age-related macular Age-Related Eye Disease Study Research Group. A randomized, placebo-controlled, clinical trial of high-dose supplementation with vitamins C and E, beta carotene, and zinc for age-related macular degeneration and vision loss: AREDS report no. 8. Arch Ophthalmol. 2001 Oct;119(10):1417-36. doi: 10.1001/archopht.119.10.1417. Erratum in: Arch Ophthalmol. 2008 Sep;126(9):1251. PMID: 11594942; PMCID: PMC1462955.

7. Age-Related Eye Disease Study 2 Research Group. Lutein + zeaxanthin and omega-3 fatty acids for age-related macular degeneration: the Age-Related Eye Disease Study 2 (AREDS2) randomized clinical trial. JAMA. 2013 May 15;309(19):2005-15. doi: 10.1001/jama.2013.4997. Erratum in: JAMA. 2013 Jul 10;310(2):208. PMID: 23644932.

8. Age-Related Eye Disease Study 2 (AREDS2) Research Group, Chew EY, SanGiovanni JP, Ferris FL, Wong WT, Agron E, Clemons TE, Sperduto R, Danis R, Chandra SR, Blodi BA, Domalpally A, Elman MJ, Antoszyk AN, Ruby AJ, Orth D, Bressler SB, Fish GE, Hubbard GB, Klein ML, Friberg TR, Rosenfeld PJ, Toth CA, Bernstein P. Lutein/zeaxanthin for the treatment of age-related cataract: AREDS2 randomized trial report no. 4. JAMA Ophthalmol. 2013 Jul;131(7):843-50. doi: 10.1001/jamaophthalmol.2013.4412. PMID: 23645227; PMCID: PMC6774801.

9. Age-Related Eye Disease Study Research Group, SanGiovanni JP, Chew EY, Clemons TE, Ferris FL 3rd, Gensler G, Lindblad AS, Milton RC, Seddon JM, Sperduto RD. The relationship of dietary carotenoid and vitamin A, E, and C intake with age-related macular degeneration in a case-control study: AREDS Report No. 22. Arch Ophthalmol. 2007 Sep;125(9):1225-32. doi: 10.1001/archopht.125.9.1225. PMID: 17846363.

10. Agrón E, Mares J, Clemons TE, Swaroop A, Chew EY, Keenan TDL; AREDS and AREDS2 Research Groups. Dietary Nutrient Intake and Progression to Late Age-Related Macular Degeneration in the Age-Related Eye Disease Studies 1 and 2. Ophthalmology. 2021 Mar;128(3):425-442. doi: 10.1016/j.ophtha.2020.08.018. Epub 2020 Aug 25. PMID: 32858063; PMCID: PMC7902480.

11. Ahmed W, Rashid S. Functional and therapeutic potential of inulin: A comprehensive review. Crit Rev Food Sci Nutr. 2019;59(1):1-13. doi: 10.1080/10408398.2017.1355775. Epub 2017 Oct 11. PMID: 28799777.

12. Ahn YJ, Kim H. Lutein as a Modulator of Oxidative Stress-Mediated Inflammatory Diseases. Antioxidants (Basel). 2021 Sep 13;10(9):1448. doi: 10.3390/antiox10091448. PMID: 34573081; PMCID: PMC8470349.

13. Alasalvar C, Chang SK, Bolling B, Oh WY, Shahidi F. Specialty seeds: Nutrients, bioactives, bioavailability, and health benefits: A comprehensive review. Compr Rev Food Sci Food Saf. 2021 May;20(3):2382-2427. doi: 10.1111/1541-4337.12730. Epub 2021 Mar 14. PMID: 33719194.

14. Alharazi WZ, McGowen A, Rose P, Jethwa PH. Could consumption of yam (Dioscorea) or its extract be beneficial in controlling glycaemia: a systematic review. Br J Nutr. 2021 Sep 15;128(4):1-12. doi: 10.1017/S0007114521003706. Epub ahead of print. PMID: 34521490; PMCID: PMC9346617.

15. Al Mahmood AM, Al-Swailem SA. Essential fatty acids in the treatment of dry eye syndrome: A myth or reality? Saudi J Ophthalmol. 2014 Jul;28(3):195-7. doi: 10.1016/j.sjopt.2014.06.004. Epub 2014 Jun 24. PMID: 25278796; PMCID: PMC4181435.

16. Al Owaifeer AM, Al Taisan AA. The Role of Diet in Glaucoma: A Review of the Current Evidence. Ophthalmol Ther. 2018 Jun;7(1):19-31. doi: 10.1007/s40123-018-0120-3. Epub 2018 Feb 8. PMID: 29423897; PMCID: PMC5997592.

17. Amirul Islam FM, Chong EW, Hodge AM, Guymer RH, Aung KZ, Makeyeva GA, Baird PN, Hopper JL, English DR, Giles GG, Robman LD. Dietary patterns and their associations with age-related macular degeneration: the Melbourne collaborative cohort study. Ophthalmology. 2014 Jul;121(7):1428-1434.e2. doi: 10.1016/j.ophtha.2014.01.002. Epub 2014 Feb 20. PMID: 24560564.

18. Aragona P, Baudouin C, Benitez Del Castillo JM, Messmer E, Barabino S, Merayo-Lloves J, Brignole-Baudouin F, Inferrera L, Rolando M, Mencucci R, Rescigno M, Bonini S, Labetoulle M. The ocular microbiome and microbiota and their effects on ocular surface pathophysiology and disorders. Surv Ophthalmol. 2021 Nov-Dec;66(6):907-925. doi: 10.1016/j.survophthal.2021.03.010. Epub 2021 Apr 2. PMID: 33819460.

19. Armstrong LE, Johnson EC. Water Intake, Water Balance, and the Elusive Daily Water Requirement. Nutrients. 2018 Dec 5;10(12):1928. doi: 10.3390/nu10121928. PMID: 30563134; PMCID: PMC6315424.

20. Arunkumar R, Gorusupudi A, Bernstein PS. The macular carotenoids: A biochemical overview. Biochim Biophys Acta Mol Cell Biol Lipids. 2020 Nov;1865(11):158617. doi: 10.1016/j.bbalip.2020.158617. Epub 2020 Jan 10. PMID: 31931175; PMCID: PMC7347445.

21. Aslam T, Delcourt C, Silva R, Holz FG, Leys A, Garcìa Layana A, Souied E. Micronutrients in age-related macular degeneration. Ophthalmologica. 2013;229(2):75-9. doi: 10.1159/000343708. Epub 2012 Nov 20. PMID: 23171595.

22. Augood C, Chakravarthy U, Young I, Vioque J, de Jong PT, Bentham G, Rahu M, Seland J, Soubrane G, Tomazzoli L, Topouzis F, Vingerling JR, Fletcher AE. Oily fish consumption, dietary docosahexaenoic acid and eicosapentaenoic acid intakes, and associations with neovascular age-related macular degeneration. Am J Clin Nutr. 2008 Aug;88(2):398-406. doi: 10.1093/ajcn/88.2.398. PMID: 18689376.

23. Awh CC, Hawken S, Zanke BW. Treatment response to antioxidants and zinc based on CFH and ARMS2 genetic risk allele number in the Age-Related Eye Disease Study. Ophthalmology. 2015 Jan;122(1):162-9. doi: 10.1016/j.ophtha.2014.07.049. Epub 2014 Sep 4. PMID: 25200399.

24. Batiha GE, Beshbishy AM, Ikram M, Mulla ZS, El-Hack MEA, Taha AE, Algammal AM, Elewa YHA. The Pharmacological Activity, Biochemical Properties, and Pharmacokinetics of the Major Natural Polyphenolic Flavonoid: Quercetin. Foods. 2020 Mar 23;9(3):374. doi: 10.3390/foods9030374. PMID: 32210182; PMCID: PMC7143931.

25. Bazzano LA, Li TY, Joshipura KJ, Hu FB. Intake of fruit, vegetables, and fruit juices and risk of diabetes in women. Diabetes Care. 2008 Jul;31(7):1311-7. doi: 10.2337/dc08-0080. Epub 2008 Apr 4. PMID: 18390796; PMCID: PMC2453647.

26. Beatty S, Chakravarthy U, Nolan JM, Muldrew KA, Woodside JV, Denny F, Stevenson MR. Secondary outcomes in a clinical trial of carotenoids with coantioxidants versus placebo in early age-related macular degeneration. Ophthalmology. 2013 Mar;120(3):600-606. doi: 10.1016/j.ophtha.2012.08.040. Epub 2012 Dec 6. PMID: 23218821.

27. Bernstein PS, Li B, Vachali PP, Gorusupudi A, Shyam R, Henriksen BS, Nolan JM. Lutein, zeaxanthin, and meso-zeaxanthin: The basic and clinical science underlying carotenoid-based nutritional interventions against ocular disease. Prog Retin Eye Res. 2016 Jan;50:34-66. doi: 10.1016/j.preteyeres.2015.10.003. Epub 2015 Nov 2. PMID: 26541886; PMCID: PMC4698241.

28. Berson EL. Nutrition and retinal degenerations. Int Ophthalmol Clin. 2000 Fall;40(4):93-111. doi: 10.1097/00004397-200010000-00008. PMID: 11064860.

29. Bird JK, Murphy RA, Ciappio ED, McBurney MI. Risk of Deficiency in Multiple Concurrent Micronutrients in Children and Adults in the United States. Nutrients. 2017 Jun 24;9(7):655. doi: 10.3390/nu9070655. PMID: 28672791; PMCID: PMC5537775.

30. Blanco-Díaz MT, Del Río-Celestino M, Martínez-Valdivieso D, Font R. Use of visible and near-infrared spectroscopy for predicting antioxidant compounds in summer squash (Cucurbita pepo ssp pepo). Food Chem. 2014 Dec 1;164:301-8. doi: 10.1016/j.foodchem.2014.05.019. Epub 2014 May 15. PMID: 24996338.

31. Blando F, Calabriso N, Berland H, Maiorano G, Gerardi C, Carluccio MA, Andersen ØM. Radical Scavenging and Anti-Inflammatory Activities of Representative Anthocyanin Groupings from Pigment-Rich Fruits and Vegetables. Int J Mol Sci. 2018 Jan 6;19(1):169. doi: 10.3390/ijms19010169. PMID: 29316619; PMCID: PMC5796118.

32. Bola C, Bartlett H, Eperjesi F. Resveratrol and the eye: activity and molecular mechanisms. Graefes Arch Clin Exp Ophthalmol. 2014 May;252(5):699-713. doi: 10.1007/s00417-014-2604-8. Epub 2014 Mar 21. PMID: 24652235.

33. Bolling BW, McKay DL, Blumberg JB. The phytochemical composition and antioxidant actions of tree nuts. Asia Pac J Clin Nutr. 2010;19(1):117-23. PMID: 20199996; PMCID: PMC5012104.

34. Bone RA, Landrum JT, Friedes LM, Gomez CM, Kilburn MD, Menendez E, Vidal I, Wang W. Distribution of lutein and zeaxanthin stereoisomers in the human retina. Exp Eye Res. 1997 Feb;64(2):211-8. doi: 10.1006/exer.1996.0210. PMID: 9176055.

35. Braakhuis A, Raman R, Vaghefi E. The Association between Dietary Intake of Antioxidants and Ocular Disease. Diseases. 2017 Jan 30;5(1):3. doi: 10.3390/diseases5010003. PMID: 28933356; PMCID: PMC5456332.

36. Brignole-Baudouin F, Baudouin C, Aragona P, Rolando M, Labetoulle M, Pisella PJ, Barabino S, Siou-Mermet R, Creuzot-Garcher C. A multicentre, double-masked, randomized, controlled trial assessing the effect of oral supplementation of omega-3 and omega-6 fatty acids on a conjunctival inflammatory marker in dry eye patients. Acta Ophthalmol. 2011 Nov;89(7):e591-7. doi: 10.1111/j.1755-3768.2011.02196.x. Epub 2011 Aug 11. PMID: 21834921.

37. Brown L, Rimm EB, Seddon JM, Giovannucci EL, Chasan-Taber L, Spiegelman D, Willett WC, Hankinson SE. A prospective study of carotenoid intake and risk of cataract extraction in US men. Am J Clin Nutr. 1999 Oct;70(4):517-24. doi: 10.1093/ajcn/70.4.517. PMID: 10500021.

38. Bulló M, Juanola-Falgarona M, Hernández-Alonso P, Salas-Salvadó J. Nutrition attributes and health effects of pistachio nuts. Br J Nutr. 2015 Apr;113 Suppl 2:S79-93. doi: 10.1017/S0007114514003250. PMID: 26148925.

39. Bungau S, Abdel-Daim MM, Tit DM, Ghanem E, Sato S, Maruyama-Inoue M, Yamane S, Kadonosono K. Health Benefits of Polyphenols and Carotenoids in Age-Related Eye Diseases. Oxid Med Cell Longev. 2019 Feb 12;2019:9783429. doi: 10.1155/2019/9783429. PMID: 30891116; PMCID: PMC6390265.

40. Calder PC. n-3 polyunsaturated fatty acids, inflammation, and inflammatory diseases. Am J Clin Nutr. 2006 Jun;83(6 Suppl):1505S-1519S. doi: 10.1093/ajcn/83.6.1505S. PMID: 16841861.

41. Cardoso, B. R., Duarte, G. B. S., Reis, B. Z., & Cozzolino, S. M. (2017). Brazil nuts: Nutritional composition, health benefits and safety aspects. Food Research International, 100, 9-18. https://doi.org/10.1016/j.foodres.2017.08.036 Cardwell G, Bornman JF, James AP, Black LJ. A Review of Mushrooms as a Potential Source of Dietary Vitamin D. Nutrients. 2018 Oct 13;10(10):1498. doi: 10.3390/nu10101498. PMID: 30322118; PMCID: PMC6213178.

42. Carneiro Â, Andrade JP. Nutritional and Lifestyle Interventions for Age-Related Macular Degeneration: A Review. Oxid Med Cell Longev. 2017;2017:6469138. doi: 10.1155/2017/6469138. Epub 2017 Jan 5. Erratum in: Oxid Med Cell Longev. 2017;2017:2435963. PMID: 28154734; PMCID: PMC5244028.

43. Carpentier S, Knaus M, Suh M. Associations between lutein, zeaxanthin, and age-related macular degeneration: an overview. Crit Rev Food Sci Nutr. 2009 Apr;49(4):313-26. doi: 10.1080/10408390802066979. PMID: 19234943.

44. Cazzola R, Della Porta M, Manoni M, Iotti S, Pinotti L, Maier JA. Going to the roots of reduced magnesium dietary intake: A tradeoff between climate changes and sources. Heliyon. 2020 Nov 3;6(11):e05390. doi: 10.1016/j.heliyon.2020.e05390. PMID: 33204877; PMCID: PMC7649274.

45. Cerino P, Buonerba C, Cannazza G, D'Auria J, Ottoni E, Fulgione A, Di Stasio A, Pierri B, Gallo A. A Review of Hemp as Food and Nutritional Supplement. Cannabis Cannabinoid Res. 2021 Feb 12;6(1):19-27. doi: 10.1089/can.2020.0001. PMID: 33614949; PMCID: PMC7891210.

46. Chan HN, Zhang XJ, Ling XT, Bui CH, Wang YM, Ip P, Chu WK, Chen LJ, Tham CC, Yam JC, Pang CP. Vitamin D and Ocular Diseases: A Systematic Review. Int J Mol Sci. 2022 Apr 11;23(8):4226. doi: 10.3390/ijms23084226. PMID: 35457041; PMCID: PMC9032397.

47. Chasan-Taber L, Willett WC, Seddon JM, Stampfer MJ, Rosner B, Colditz GA, Speizer FE, Hankinson SE. A prospective study of carotenoid and vitamin A intakes and risk of cataract extraction in US women. Am J Clin Nutr. 1999 Oct;70(4):509-16. doi: 10.1093/ajcn/70.4.509. PMID: 10500020.

48. Chaudhry S, Dunn H, Carnt N, White A. Nutritional supplementation in the prevention and treatment of glaucoma. Surv Ophthalmol. 2022 Jul-Aug;67(4):1081-1098. doi: 10.1016/j.survophthal.2021.12.001. Epub 2021 Dec 8. PMID: 34896192.

49. Chen CY, Milbury PE, Chung SK, Blumberg J. Effect of almond skin polyphenolics and quercetin on human LDL and apolipoprotein B-100 oxidation and conformation. J Nutr Biochem. 2007 Dec;18(12):785-94. doi: 10.1016/j.jnutbio.2006.12.015. Epub 2007 May 2. PMID: 17475462.

50. Chen N, Bezzina R, Hinch E, Lewandowski PA, Cameron-Smith D, Mathai ML, Jois M, Sinclair AJ, Begg DP, Wark JD, Weisinger HS, Weisinger RS. Green tea, black tea, and epigallocatechin modify body composition, improve glucose tolerance, and differentially alter metabolic gene expression in rats fed a high-fat diet. Nutr Res. 2009 Nov;29(11):784-93. doi: 10.1016/j.nutres.2009.10.003. PMID: 19932867.

51. Chen SJ, Lee CJ, Lin TB, Peng HY, Liu HJ, Chen YS, Tseng KW. Protective Effects of Fucoxanthin on Ultraviolet B-Induced Corneal Denervation and Inflammatory Pain in a Rat Model. Mar Drugs. 2019 Mar 5;17(3):152. doi: 10.3390/md17030152. PMID: 30841522; PMCID: PMC6471339.

52. Chen SJ, Lee CJ, Lin TB, Liu HJ, Huang SY, Chen JZ, Tseng KW. Inhibition of Ultraviolet B-Induced Expression of the Proinflammatory Cytokines TNF-α and VEGF in the Cornea by Fucoxanthin Treatment in a Rat Model. Mar Drugs. 2016 Jan 7;14(1):13. doi: 10.3390/md14010013. PMID: 26751458; PMCID: PMC4728510.

53. Chen W, Ye Y, Wu Z, Lin J, Wang Y, Ding Q, Yang X, Yang W, Lin B, Lin B. Temporary Upregulation of Nrf2 by Naringenin Alleviates Oxidative Damage in the Retina and ARPE-19 Cells. Oxid Med Cell Longev. 2021 Nov 17;2021:4053276. doi: 10.1155/2021/4053276. PMID: 34840667; PMCID: PMC8612781.

54. Chew EY, Clemons TE, Agrón E, Domalpally A, Keenan TDL, Vitale S, Weber C, Smith DC, Christen W; AREDS2 Research Group. Long-term Outcomes of Adding Lutein/Zeaxanthin and ω-3 Fatty Acids to the AREDS Supplements on Age-Related Macular Degeneration Progression: AREDS2 Report 28. JAMA Ophthalmol. 2022 Jul 1;140(7):692-698. doi: 10.1001/jamaophthalmol.2022.1640. PMID: 35653117; PMCID: PMC9164119.

55. Chew EY, Clemons TE, Agrón E, Sperduto RD, Sangiovanni JP, Kurinij N, Davis MD; Age-Related Eye Disease Study Research Group. Long-term effects of vitamins C and E, β-carotene, and zinc on age-related macular degeneration: AREDS report no. 35. Ophthalmology. 2013 Aug;120(8):1604-11.e4. doi: 10.1016/j.ophtha.2013.01.021. Epub 2013 Apr 10. Erratum in: Ophthalmology. 2016 Dec;123(12):2634. PMID: 23582353; PMCID: PMC3728272.

56. Chew EY. Age-related Macular Degeneration: Nutrition, Genes and Deep Learning-The LXXVI Edward Jackson Memorial Lecture. Am J Ophthalmol. 2020 Sep;217:335-347. doi: 10.1016/j.ajo.2020.05.042. Epub 2020 Jun 20. Erratum in: Am J Ophthalmol. 2021 Nov;231:212. PMID: 32574780; PMCID: PMC8324084.

57. Chew EY. Nutrition, Genes, and Age-Related Macular Degeneration: What Have We Learned from the Trials? Ophthalmologica. 2017;238(1-2):1-5. doi: 10.1159/000473865. Epub 2017 May 6. PMID: 28478452; PMCID: PMC5532061.

58. Chew EY. Vitamins and minerals, for eyes only? JAMA Ophthalmol. 2014 Jun;132(6):665-6. doi: 10.1001/jamaophthalmol.2014.643. PMID: 24651887.

59. Chitchumroonchokchai C, Schwartz SJ, Failla ML. Assessment of lutein bioavailability from meals and a supplement using simulated digestion and caco-2 human intestinal cells. J Nutr. 2004 Sep;134(9):2280-6. doi: 10.1093/jn/134.9.2280. PMID: 15333717.

60. Chiu CJ, Milton RC, Klein R, Gensler G, Taylor A. Dietary compound score and risk of age-related macular degeneration in the age-related eye disease study. Ophthalmology. 2009 May;116(5):939-46. doi: 10.1016/j.ophtha.2008.12.025. PMID: 19410952; PMCID: PMC3753024.

61. Chiu CJ, Milton RC, Klein R, Gensler G, Taylor A. Dietary carbohydrate and the progression of age-related macular degeneration: a prospective study from the Age-Related Eye Disease Study. Am J Clin Nutr. 2007 Oct;86(4):1210-8. doi: 10.1093/ajcn/86.4.1210. PMID: 17921404.

62. Chiu CJ, Chang ML, Li T, Gensler G, Taylor A. Visualization of Dietary Patterns and Their Associations With Age-Related Macular Degeneration. Invest Ophthalmol Vis Sci. 2017 Mar 1;58(3):1404-1410. doi: 10.1167/iovs.16-20454. PMID: 28253403; PMCID: PMC5361454.

63. Chiu CJ, Klein R, Milton RC, Gensler G, Taylor A. Does eating particular diets alter the risk of age-related macular degeneration in users of the Age-Related Eye Disease Study supplements? Br J Ophthalmol. 2009 Sep;93(9):1241-6. doi: 10.1136/bjo.2008.143412. Epub 2009 Jun 9. PMID: 19508997; PMCID: PMC3033729.

64. Chiu CJ, Milton RC, Gensler G, Taylor A. Association between dietary glycemic index and age-related macular degeneration in nondiabetic participants in the Age-Related Eye Disease Study. Am J Clin Nutr. 2007 Jul;86(1):180-8. doi: 10.1093/ajcn/86.1.180. PMID: 17616779.

65. Chiu CJ, Milton RC, Gensler G, Taylor A. Dietary carbohydrate intake and glycemic index in relation to cortical and nuclear lens opacities in the Age-Related Eye Disease Study. Am J Clin Nutr. 2006 May;83(5):1177-84. doi: 10.1093/ajcn/83.5.1177. PMID: 16685063.

66. Christen WG Jr. Antioxidants and eye disease. Am J Med. 1994 Sep 26;97(3A):14S-17S; discussion 22S-28S. doi: 10.1016/0002-9343(94)90293-3. PMID: 8085581.

67. Christen WG, Chasman DI, Cook NR, Chiuve SE, Ridker PM, Buring JE. Homocysteine, B Vitamins, MTHFR Genotype, and Incident Age-related Macular Degeneration. Ophthalmol Retina. 2018 May;2(5):508-510. doi: 10.1016/j.oret.2017.10.001. PMID: 29963648; PMCID: PMC6022858.

68. Cho E, Seddon JM, Rosner B, Willett WC, Hankinson SE. Prospective study of intake of fruits, vegetables, vitamins, and carotenoids and risk of age-related maculopathy. Arch Ophthalmol. 2004 Jun;122(6):883-92. doi: 10.1001/archopht.122.6.883. PMID: 15197064.

69. Cho E, Hung S, Willett WC, Spiegelman D, Rimm EB, Seddon JM, Colditz GA, Hankinson SE. Prospective study of dietary fat and the risk of age-related macular degeneration. Am J Clin Nutr. 2001 Feb;73(2):209-18. doi: 10.1093/ajcn/73.2.209. PMID: 11157315.

70. Cho E, Stampfer MJ, Seddon JM, Hung S, Spiegelman D, Rimm EB, Willett WC, Hankinson SE. Prospective study of zinc intake and the risk of age-related macular degeneration. Ann Epidemiol. 2001 Jul;11(5):328-36. doi: 10.1016/s1047-2797(01)00217-4. PMID: 11399447.

71. Chua B, Flood V, Rochtchina E, Wang JJ, Smith W, Mitchell P. Dietary fatty acids and the 5-year incidence of age-related maculopathy. Arch Ophthalmol. 2006 Jul;124(7):981-6. doi: 10.1001/archopht.124.7.981. PMID: 16832021.

72. Chucair AJ, Rotstein NP, Sangiovanni JP, During A, Chew EY, Politi LE. Lutein and zeaxanthin protect photoreceptors from apoptosis induced by oxidative stress: relation with docosahexaenoic acid. Invest Ophthalmol Vis Sci. 2007 Nov;48(11):5168-77. doi: 10.1167/iovs.07-0037. PMID: 17962470.

73. Chung HY, Rasmussen HM, Johnson EJ. Lutein bioavailability is higher from lutein-enriched eggs than from supplements and spinach in men. J Nutr. 2004 Aug;134(8):1887-93. doi: 10.1093/jn/134.8.1887. PMID: 15284371.

74. Chylack LT Jr, Brown NP, Bron A, Hurst M, Köpcke W, Thien U, Schalch W. The Roche European American Cataract Trial (REACT): a randomized clinical trial to investigate the efficacy of an oral antioxidant micronutrient mixture to slow progression of age-related cataract. Ophthalmic Epidemiol. 2002 Feb;9(1):49-80. doi: 10.1076/opep.9.1.49.1717. PMID: 11815895.

75. Cömert ED, Mogol BA, Gökmen V. Relationship between color and antioxidant capacity of fruits and vegetables. Curr Res Food Sci. 2019 Nov 21;2:1-10. doi: 10.1016/j.crfs.2019.11.001. PMID: 32914105; PMCID: PMC7473347.

76. Congdon N, O'Colmain B, Klaver CC, Klein R, Muñoz B, Friedman DS, Kempen J, Taylor HR, Mitchell P; Eye Diseases Prevalence Research Group. Causes and prevalence of visual impairment among adults in the United States. Arch Ophthalmol. 2004 Apr;122(4):477-85. doi: 10.1001/archopht.122.4.477. PMID: 15078664.

77. Connor KM, SanGiovanni JP, Lofqvist C, Aderman CM, Chen J, Higuchi A, Hong S, Pravda EA, Majchrzak S, Carper D, Hellstrom A, Kang JX, Chew EY, Salem N Jr, Serhan CN, Smith LEH. Increased dietary intake of omega-3-polyunsaturated fatty acids reduces pathological retinal angiogenesis. Nat Med. 2007 Jul;13(7):868-873. doi: 10.1038/nm1591. Epub 2007 Jun 24. PMID: 17589522; PMCID: PMC4491412.

78. Cordain L, Eaton SB, Sebastian A, Mann N, Lindeberg S, Watkins BA, O'Keefe JH, Brand-Miller J. Origins and evolution of the Western diet: health implications for the 21st century. Am J Clin Nutr. 2005 Feb;81(2):341-54. doi: 10.1093/ajcn.81.2.341. PMID: 15699220.

79. Cougnard-Grégoire A, Merle BM, Korobelnik JF, Rougier MB, Delyfer MN, Le Goff M, Samieri C, Dartigues JF, Delcourt C. Olive Oil Consumption and Age-Related Macular Degeneration: The Alienor Study. PLoS One. 2016 Jul 28;11(7):e0160240. doi: 10.1371/journal.pone.0160240. PMID: 27467382; PMCID: PMC4965131.

80. Csader S, Korhonen S, Kaarniranta K, Schwab U. The Effect of Dietary Supplementations on Delaying the Progression of Age-Related Macular Degeneration: A Systematic Review and Meta-Analysis. Nutrients. 2022 Oct 13;14(20):4273. doi: 10.3390/nu14204273. PMID: 36296956; PMCID: PMC9610847.

81. Cumming RG, Mitchell P, Smith W. Diet and cataract: the Blue Mountains Eye Study. Ophthalmology. 2000 Mar;107(3):450-6. doi: 10.1016/s0161-6420(99)00024-x. PMID: 10711880.

82. Dagnelie G, Zorge IS, McDonald TM. Lutein improves visual function in some patients with retinal degeneration: a pilot study via the Internet. Optometry. 2000 Mar;71(3):147-64. PMID: 10970259.

83. Dawe RS. Further evidence for carotenoid antioxidants in photoprotection. Br J Dermatol. 2017 May;176(5):1120-1121. doi: 10.1111/bjd.15487. PMID: 28504382.

84. Delcourt C, Carrière I, Cristol JP, Lacroux A, Gerber M. Dietary fat and the risk of age-related maculopathy: the POLANUT study. Eur J Clin Nutr. 2007 Nov;61(11):1341-4. doi: 10.1038/sj.ejcn.1602685. Epub 2007 Feb 14. PMID: 17299457.

85. Downie LE, Ng SM, Lindsley KB, Akpek EK. Omega-3 and omega-6 polyunsaturated fatty acids for dry eye disease. Cochrane Database Syst Rev. 2019 Dec 18;12(12):CD011016. doi: 10.1002/14651858.CD011016.pub2. PMID: 31847055; PMCID: PMC6917524.

86. Du W, An Y, He X, Zhang D, He W. Protection of Kaempferol on Oxidative Stress-Induced Retinal Pigment Epithelial Cell Damage. Oxid Med Cell Longev. 2018 Nov 21;2018:1610751. doi: 10.1155/2018/1610751. PMID: 30584457; PMCID: PMC6280232.

87. Dulull NK, Dias DA, Thrimawithana TR, Kwa FAA. L-Sulforaphane Confers Protection Against Oxidative Stress in an In Vitro Model of Age-Related Macular Degeneration. Curr Mol Pharmacol. 2018;11(3):237-253. doi: 10.2174/1874467211666180125163009. PMID: 29376497.

88. Dziedziak J, Kasarełło K, Cudnoch-Jędrzejewska A. Dietary Antioxidants in Age-Related Macular Degeneration and Glaucoma. Antioxidants (Basel). 2021 Oct 30;10(11):1743. doi: 10.3390/antiox10111743. PMID: 34829613; PMCID: PMC8614766.

89. Eisenhauer B, Natoli S, Liew G, Flood VM. Lutein and Zeaxanthin-Food Sources, Bioavailability and Dietary Variety in Age-Related Macular Degeneration Protection. Nutrients. 2017 Feb 9;9(2):120. doi: 10.3390/nu9020120. PMID: 28208784; PMCID: PMC5331551.

90. Elizabeth L, Machado P, Zinöcker M, Baker P, Lawrence M. Ultra-Processed Foods and Health Outcomes: A Narrative Review. Nutrients. 2020 Jun 30;12(7):1955. doi: 10.3390/nu12071955. PMID: 32630022; PMCID: PMC7399967.

91. Evans JR, Lawrenson JG. Dietary interventions for AMD: what do we know and what do we not know? Br J Ophthalmol. 2013 Sep;97(9):1089-90. doi: 10.1136/bjophthalmol-2013-303134. Epub 2013 Mar 9. PMID: 23476030.

92. Fang J. Classification of fruits based on anthocyanin types and relevance to their health effects. Nutrition. 2015 Nov-Dec;31(11-12):1301-6. doi: 10.1016/j.nut.2015.04.015. Epub 2015 May 15. PMID: 26250485.

93. Fehér J, Élő Á, István L, Nagy ZZ, Radák Z, Scuderi G, Artico M, Kovács I. Microbiota mitochondria disorders as hubs for early age-related macular degeneration. Geroscience. 2022 Aug 18:1–31. doi: 10.1007/s11357-022-00620-5. Epub ahead of print. PMID: 35978068; PMCID: PMC9385247.

94. Fernández-Sánchez L, Lax P, Noailles A, Angulo A, Maneu V, Cuenca N. Natural Compounds from Saffron and Bear Bile Prevent Vision Loss and Retinal Degeneration. Molecules. 2015 Jul 31;20(8):13875-93. doi: 10.3390/molecules200813875. PMID: 26263962; PMCID: PMC6332441.

95. Ferretti G, Bacchetti T, Belleggia A, Neri D. Cherry antioxidants: from farm to table. Molecules. 2010 Oct 12;15(10):6993-7005. doi: 10.3390/molecules15106993. PMID: 20944519; PMCID: PMC6259571.

96. Fletcher AE, Bentham GC, Agnew M, Young IS, Augood C, Chakravarthy U, de Jong PT, Rahu M, Seland J, Soubrane G, Tomazzoli L, Topouzis F, Vingerling JR, Vioque J. Sunlight exposure, antioxidants, and age-related macular degeneration. Arch Ophthalmol. 2008 Oct;126(10):1396-403. doi: 10.1001/archopht.126.10.1396. PMID: 18852418.

97. Flood VM, Burlutsky G, Webb KL, Wang JJ, Smith WT, Mitchell P. Food and nutrient consumption trends in older Australians: a 10-year cohort study. Eur J Clin Nutr. 2010 Jun;64(6):603-13. doi: 10.1038/ejcn.2010.34. Epub 2010 Mar 17. PMID: 20234384.

98. Fung TT, Hu FB, Pereira MA, Liu S, Stampfer MJ, Colditz GA, Willett WC. Whole-grain intake and the risk of type 2 diabetes: a prospective study in men. Am J Clin Nutr. 2002 Sep;76(3):535-40. doi: 10.1093/ajcn/76.3.535. PMID: 12197996.

99. García-Marqués JV, Talens-Estarelles C, García-Lázaro S, Wolffsohn JS, Cerviño A. Systemic, environmental and lifestyle risk factors for dry eye disease in a mediterranean caucasian population. Cont Lens Anterior Eye. 2022 Oct;45(5):101539. doi: 10.1016/j.clae.2021.101539. Epub 2021 Nov 14. PMID: 34789408.

100. Garrido I, Monagas M, Gómez-Cordovés C, Bartolomé B. Polyphenols and antioxidant properties of almond skins: influence of industrial processing. J Food Sci. 2008 Mar;73(2):C106-15. doi: 10.1111/j.1750-3841.2007.00637.x. PMID: 18298714.

101. Glaser TS, Doss LE, Shih G, Nigam D, Sperduto RD, Ferris FL 3rd, Agrón E, Clemons TE, Chew EY; Age-Related Eye Disease Study Research Group. The Association of Dietary Lutein plus Zeaxanthin and B Vitamins with Cataracts in the Age-Related Eye Disease Study: AREDS Report No. 37. Ophthalmology. 2015 Jul;122(7):1471-9. doi: 10.1016/j.ophtha.2015.04.007. Epub 2015 May 9. PMID: 25972257; PMCID: PMC4485544.

102. Gopinath B, Liew G, Tang D, Burlutsky G, Flood VM, Mitchell P. Consumption of eggs and the 15-year incidence of age-related macular degeneration. Clin Nutr. 2020 Feb;39(2):580-584. doi: 10.1016/j.clnu.2019.03.009. Epub 2019 Mar 16. PMID: 30914217.

103. Gopinath B, Liew G, Kifley A, Flood VM, Joachim N, Lewis JR, Hodgson JM, Mitchell P. Dietary flavonoids and the prevalence and 15-y incidence of age-related macular degeneration. Am J Clin Nutr. 2018 Aug 1;108(2):381-387. doi: 10.1093/ajcn/nqy114. PMID: 29982448.

104. Gopinath B, Flood VM, Louie JC, Wang JJ, Burlutsky G, Rochtchina E, Mitchell P. Consumption of dairy products and the 15-year incidence of age-related macular degeneration. Br J Nutr. 2014 May;111(9):1673-9. doi: 10.1017/S000711451300408X. Epub 2014 Feb 6. PMID: 24502821.

105. Gopinath B, Flood VM, Rochtchina E, Wang JJ, Mitchell P. Homocysteine, folate, vitamin B-12, and 10-y incidence of age-related macular degeneration. Am J Clin Nutr. 2013 Jul;98(1):129-35. doi: 10.3945/ajcn.112.057091. Epub 2013 May 1. PMID: 23636242.

106. Goyal A, Tanwar B, Kumar Sihag M, Sharma V. Sacha inchi (Plukenetia volubilis L.): An emerging source of nutrients, omega-3 fatty acid and phytochemicals. Food Chem. 2022 Mar 30;373(Pt B):131459. doi: 10.1016/j.foodchem.2021.131459. Epub 2021 Oct 23. PMID: 34731811.

107. Grotto D, Zied E. The Standard American Diet and its relationship to the health status of Americans. Nutr Clin Pract. 2010 Dec;25(6):603-12. doi: 10.1177/0884533610386234. PMID: 21139124.

108. Gujral GS, Askari SN, Ahmad S, Zakir SM, Saluja K. Topical vitamin C, vitamin E, and acetylcysteine as corneal wound healing agents: A comparative study. Indian J Ophthalmol. 2020 Dec;68(12):2935-2939. doi: 10.4103/ijo.IJO_1463_20. PMID: 33229673; PMCID: PMC7856962.

109. Halvorsen BL, Carlsen MH, Phillips KM, Bøhn SK, Holte K, Jacobs DR Jr, Blomhoff R. Content of redox-active compounds (ie, antioxidants) in foods consumed in the United States. Am J Clin Nutr. 2006 Jul;84(1):95-135. doi: 10.1093/ajcn/84.1.95. PMID: 16825686.

110. Hankinson SE, Stampfer MJ, Seddon JM, Colditz GA, Rosner B, Speizer FE, Willett WC. Nutrient intake and cataract extraction in women: a prospective study. BMJ. 1992 Aug 8;305(6849):335-9. doi: 10.1136/bmj.305.6849.335. PMID: 1392884; PMCID: PMC1882980.

111. Hashem HE, Abd El-Haleem MR, Amer MG, Bor'i A. Pomegranate protective effect on experimental ischemia/reperfusion retinal injury in rats (histological and biochemical study). Ultrastruct Pathol. 2017 Sep-Oct;41(5):346-357. doi: 10.1080/01913123.2017.1346737. Epub 2017 Aug 10. PMID: 28796566.

112. Health Benefits. *The Health Benefits of Xigua Fruit.* Available at: https://healthybenefits.info/the-health-benefits-of-xigua-fruit/. Accessed June 30, 2022.

113. Healthline. 7 Surprising Health Benefits of Eating Seaweed. Available at: https://www.healthline.com/nutrition/benefits-of-seaweed. Accessed June 15, 2022.

114. Healthline. 7 Science-Based Health Benefits of Drinking Enough Water. Available at: https://www.healthline.com/nutrition/7-health-benefits-of-water. Accessed June 15, 2022.

115. Healthline. 7 Benefits of Purple Yam (Ube), and How It Differs from Taro. Available at: https://www.healthline.com/nutrition/ube-purple-yam.Accessed June 30, 2022.

116. Healthline. 8 Science-Backed Benefits of Paprika. Available at: https://www.healthline.com/nutrition/paprika-benefits. Accessed June 14, 2022.

117. Healthline. 8 Evidence-Based Health Benefits of Quinoa. Available at: https://www.healthline.com/nutrition/8-health-benefits-quinoa. Accessed June 15, 2022.

118. Healthline. *8 Impressive Health Benefits and Uses of Parsley.* Available at: https://www.healthline.com/nutrition/parsley-benefits. Accessed June 14, 2022.

119. Healthline. *9 Health Benefits of Pistachios.* Available at: https://www.healthline.com/nutrition/9-benefits-of-pistachios. Accessed June 14, 2022.

120. Healthline. *11 Health and Nutrition Benefits of Yams.* Available at: https://www.healthline.com/nutrition/yam-benefits. Accessed June 30, 2022.

121. Healthline. *12 Health and Nutrition Benefits of Zucchini.* Available at: https://www.healthline.com/nutrition/zucchini-benefits. Accessed June 30, 2022.

122. Healthline. *Are Mushrooms Good For You?* Available at: https://www.healthline.com/health/food-nutrition/are-mushrooms-good-for-you. Accessed 7-30-2022.

123. Healthline. *Does Flaxseed Oil treat Dry Eyes?* Available at: https://www.healthline.com/health/dry-eye/flaxseed-oil-for-dry-eyes. Accessed June 4, 2022.

124. Healthline. *Four Health Benefits of Kiwi.* Available at: https://www.healthline.com/nutrition/kiwi-benefits#Kiwi-benefits. Accessed 7-20-2022.

125. Healthline. *Onions 101: Nutrition Facts and Health Effects.* Available at: https://www.healthline.com/nutrition/foods/onions#plant-compounds. Accessed 7-20-2022.

126. Healthline. *Pomegranate: 10 Health and Nutritional Benefits.* Available at: https://www.healthline.com/nutrition/12-proven-benefits-of-pomegranate. Accessed June 15, 2022.

127. Healthline.*Tomatoes 101: Nutrition Facts and Health Benefits.* Available at: https://www.healthline.com/nutrition/foods/tomatoes. Accessed June 15, 2022.

128. Healthline. *What Is Ugli Fruit? Everything You Need to Know.* Available at: https://www.healthline.com/nutrition/ugli-fruit. Accessed June 29, 2022.

129. Healthline. The Top 9 Health Benefits of Watermelon. Available at: https://www.healthline.com/nutrition/watermelon-health-benefits. Accessed June 30, 2022.

130. Hu FB, Manson JE, Stampfer MJ, Colditz G, Liu S, Solomon CG, Willett WC. Diet, lifestyle, and the risk of type 2 diabetes mellitus in women. N Engl J Med. 2001 Sep 13;345(11):790-7. doi: 10.1056/NEJMoa010492. PMID: 11556298.

131. Jacques PF, Chylack LT Jr, Hankinson SE, Khu PM, Rogers G, Friend J, Tung W, Wolfe JK, Padhye N, Willett WC, Taylor A. Long-term nutrient intake and early age-related nuclear lens opacities. Arch Ophthalmol. 2001 Jul;119(7):1009-19. doi: 10.1001/archopht.119.7.1009. PMID: 11448323.

132. Jacques PF, Taylor A, Hankinson SE, Willett WC, Mahnken B, Lee Y, Vaid K, Lahav M. Long-term vitamin C supplement use and prevalence of early age-related lens opacities. Am J Clin Nutr. 1997 Oct;66(4):911-6. doi: 10.1093/ajcn/66.4.911. PMID: 9322567.

133. Jannasch F, Kröger J, Schulze MB. Dietary Patterns and Type 2 Diabetes: A Systematic Literature Review and Meta-Analysis of Prospective Studies. J Nutr. 2017 Jun;147(6):1174-1182. doi: 10.3945/jn.116.242552. Epub 2017 Apr 19. PMID: 28424256.

134. Järvinen RL, Larmo PS, Setälä NL, Yang B, Engblom JR, Viitanen MH, Kallio HP. Effects of oral sea buckthorn oil on tear film Fatty acids in individuals with dry eye. Cornea. 2011 Sep;30(9):1013-9. doi: 10.1097/ICO.0b013e3182035ad9. PMID: 21832964.

135. Jenkins DJ, Kendall CW, Augustin LS, Franceschi S, Hamidi M, Marchie A, Jenkins AL, Axelsen M. Glycemic index: overview of implications in health and disease. Am J Clin Nutr. 2002 Jul;76(1):266S-73S. doi: 10.1093/ajcn/76/1.266S. PMID: 12081850.

136. Jenkins DJ, Kendall CW, Josse AR, Salvatore S, Brighenti F, Augustin LS, Ellis PR, Vidgen E, Rao AV. Almonds decrease postprandial glycemia, insulinemia, and oxidative damage in healthy individuals. J Nutr. 2006 Dec;136(12):2987-92. doi: 10.1093/jn/136.12.2987. PMID: 17116708.

137. Jia YP, Sun L, Yu HS, Liang LP, Li W, Ding H, Song XB, Zhang LJ. The Pharmacological Effects of Lutein and Zeaxanthin on Visual Disorders and Cognition Diseases. Molecules. 2017 Apr 20;22(4):610. doi: 10.3390/molecules22040610. PMID: 28425969; PMCID: PMC6154331.

138. Johnson EJ, Schaefer EJ. Potential role of dietary n-3 fatty acids in the prevention of dementia and macular degeneration. Am J Clin Nutr. 2006 Jun;83(6 Suppl):1494S-1498S. doi: 10.1093/ajcn/83.6.1494S. Erratum in: Am J Clin Nutr. 2006 Dec;84(6):1555. PMID: 16841859.

139. Johra FT, Bepari AK, Bristy AT, Reza HM. A Mechanistic Review of β-Carotene, Lutein, and Zeaxanthin in Eye Health and Disease. Antioxidants (Basel). 2020 Oct 26;9(11):1046. doi: 10.3390/antiox9111046. PMID: 33114699; PMCID: PMC7692753.c

140. Kao YW, Hsu SK, Chen JY, Lin IL, Chen KJ, Lee PY, Ng HS, Chiu CC, Cheng KC. Curcumin Metabolite Tetrahydrocurcumin in the Treatment of Eye Diseases. Int J Mol Sci. 2020 Dec 28;22(1):212. doi: 10.3390/ijms22010212. PMID: 33379248; PMCID: PMC7795090.

141. Katsirma Z, Dimidi E, Rodriguez-Mateos A, Whelan K. Fruits and their impact on the gut microbiota, gut motility and constipation. Food Funct. 2021 Oct 4;12(19):8850-8866. doi: 10.1039/d1fo01125a. PMID: 34505614.

142. Kim KA, Kim SM, Kang SW, Jeon SI, Um BH, Jung SH. Edible seaweed, Eisenia bicyclis, protects retinal ganglion cells death caused by oxidative stress. Mar Biotechnol (NY). 2012 Aug;14(4):383-95. doi: 10.1007/s10126-012-9459-y. Epub 2012 May 18. PMID: 22610700.

143. Kimura Y, Mori D, Imada T, Izuta Y, Shibuya M, Sakaguchi H, Oonishi E, Okada N, Matsumoto K, Tsubota K. Restoration of Tear Secretion in a Murine Dry Eye Model by Oral Administration of Palmitoleic Acid. Nutrients. 2017 Apr 5;9(4):364. doi: 10.3390/nu9040364. PMID: 28379171; PMCID: PMC5409703.

144. Kwa FA, Dulull NK, Roessner U, Dias DA, Rupasinghe TW. Lipidomics reveal the protective effects of a vegetable-derived isothiocyanate against retinal degeneration. F1000Res. 2019 Jul 12;8:1067. doi: 10.12688/f1000research.19598.5. PMID: 33145006; PMCID: PMC7590896.

145. Lacka K, Szeliga A. Significance of selenium in thyroid physiology and pathology. Pol Merkur Lekarski. 2015 Jun;38(228):348-53. PMID: 26098657.

146. Larmo PS, Järvinen RL, Setälä NL, Yang B, Viitanen MH, Engblom JR, Tahvonen RL, Kallio HP. Oral sea buckthorn oil attenuates tear film osmolarity and symptoms in individuals with dry eye. J Nutr. 2010 Aug;140(8):1462-8. doi: 10.3945/jn.109.118901. Epub 2010 Jun 16. PMID: 20554904.

147. Lawrenson JG, Downie LE. Nutrition and Eye Health. Nutrients. 2019 Sep 6;11(9):2123. doi: 10.3390/nu11092123. PMID: 31489894; PMCID: PMC6771137.

148. Layana AG, Minnella AM, Garhöfer G, Aslam T, Holz FG, Leys A, Silva R, Delcourt C, Souied E, Seddon JM. Vitamin D and Age-Related Macular Degeneration. Nutrients. 2017 Oct 13;9(10):1120. doi: 10.3390/nu9101120. PMID: 29027953; PMCID: PMC5691736.

149. Lenzi Q, Correia-Santos AM, Lenzi-Almeida KC, Boaventura GT. Flaxseed used since pregnancy by the mother and after weaning by the offspring benefits the retina and optic nerve development in rats. J Matern Fetal Neonatal Med. 2018 Mar;31(5):625-632. doi: 10.1080/14767058.2017.1293028. Epub 2017 Feb 28. PMID: 28282776.

150. Li J, Yip YWY, Ren J, Hui WK, He JN, Yu QX, Chu KO, Ng TK, Chan SO, Pang CP, Chu WK. Green tea catechins alleviate autoimmune symptoms and visual impairment in a murine model for human chronic intraocular inflammation by inhibiting Th17-associated pro-inflammatory gene expression. Sci Rep. 2019 Feb 19;9(1):2301. doi: 10.1038/s41598-019-38868-1. PMID: 30783194; PMCID: PMC6381204.

151. Li L, Geng X, Tian L, Wang D, Wang Q. Grape seed proanthocyanidins protect retinal ganglion cells by inhibiting oxidative stress and mitochondrial alteration. Arch Pharm Res. 2020 Oct;43(10):1056-1066. doi: 10.1007/s12272-020-01272-9. Epub 2020 Oct 19. PMID: 33078305.

152. Li N, Wu X, Zhuang W, Xia L, Chen Y, Wang Y, Wu C, Rao Z, Du L, Zhao R, Yi M, Wan Q, Zhou Y. Green leafy vegetable and lutein intake and multiple health outcomes. Food Chem. 2021 Oct 30;360:130145. doi: 10.1016/j.foodchem.2021.130145. Epub 2021 May 18. PMID: 34034049.

153. Li N, Jia X, Chen CY, Blumberg JB, Song Y, Zhang W, Zhang X, Ma G, Chen J. Almond consumption reduces oxidative DNA damage and lipid peroxidation in male smokers. J Nutr. 2007 Dec;137(12):2717-22. doi: 10.1093/jn/137.12.2717. PMID: 18029489.

154. Li T , Chen L , Xiao J , An F , Wan C , Song H . Prebiotic effects of resistant starch from purple yam (Dioscorea alata L.) on the tolerance and proliferation ability of Bifidobacterium adolescentis in vitro. Food Funct. 2018 Apr 25;9(4):2416-2425. doi: 10.1039/c7fo01919j. PMID: 29620784.

155. Lim JC, Caballero Arredondo M, Braakhuis AJ, Donaldson PJ. Vitamin C and the Lens: New Insights into Delaying the Onset of Cataract. Nutrients. 2020 Oct 14;12(10):3142. doi: 10.3390/nu12103142. PMID: 33066702; PMCID: PMC7602486.

156. Lin M, Han P, Li Y, Wang W, Lai D, Zhou L. Quinoa Secondary Metabolites and Their Biological Activities or Functions. Molecules. 2019 Jul 9;24(13):2512. doi: 10.3390/molecules24132512. PMID: 31324047; PMCID: PMC6651730.

157. Lister T. Nutritional, Alternative, and Complementary Therapies for Age-related Macular Degeneration. Integr Med (Encinitas). 2019 Dec;18(6):30-36. PMID: 32549854; PMCID: PMC7238905.

158. Liu R, Wang T, Zhang B, Qin L, Wu C, Li Q, Ma L. Lutein and zeaxanthin supplementation and association with visual function in age-related macular degeneration. Invest Ophthalmol Vis Sci. 2014 Dec 16;56(1):252-8. doi: 10.1167/iovs.14-15553. PMID: 25515572.

159. Liu XH, Yu RB, Liu R, Hao ZX, Han CC, Zhu ZH, Ma L. Association between lutein and zeaxanthin status and the risk of cataract: a meta-analysis. Nutrients. 2014 Jan 22;6(1):452-65. doi: 10.3390/nu6010452. PMID: 24451312; PMCID: PMC3916871.

160. Liu XF, Hao JL, Xie T, Mukhtar NJ, Zhang W, Malik TH, Lu CW, Zhou DD. Curcumin, A Potential Therapeutic Candidate for Anterior Segment Eye Diseases: A Review. Front Pharmacol. 2017 Feb 14;8:66. doi: 10.3389/fphar.2017.00066. PMID: 28261099; PMCID: PMC5306202.

161. Llop SM, Davoudi S, Stanwyck LK, Sathe S, Tom L, Ahmadi T, Grotting L, Papaliodis GN, Sobrin L. Association of Low Vitamin D Levels with Noninfectious Uveitis and Scleritis. Ocul Immunol Inflamm. 2019;27(4):602-609. doi: 10.1080/09273948.2018.1434208. Epub 2018 Feb 23. PMID: 29474126.

162. Ma L, Hao ZX, Liu RR, Yu RB, Shi Q, Pan JP. A dose-response meta-analysis of dietary lutein and zeaxanthin intake in relation to risk of age-related cataract. Graefes Arch Clin Exp Ophthalmol. 2014 Jan;252(1):63-70. doi: 10.1007/s00417-013-2492-3. Epub 2013 Oct 23. PMID: 24150707.

163. Mahmassani HA, Avendano EE, Raman G, Johnson EJ. Avocado consumption and risk factors for heart disease: a systematic review and meta-analysis. Am J Clin Nutr. 2018 Apr 1;107(4):523-536. doi: 10.1093/ajcn/nqx078. PMID: 29635493.

164. Mares J. Lutein and Zeaxanthin Isomers in Eye Health and Disease. Annu Rev Nutr. 2016 Jul 17;36:571-602. doi: 10.1146/annurev-nutr-071715-051110. PMID: 27431371; PMCID: PMC5611842.

165. Mares JA, LaRowe TL, Snodderly DM, Moeller SM, Gruber MJ, Klein ML, Wooten BR, Johnson EJ, Chappell RJ; CAREDS Macular Pigment Study Group and Investigators. Predictors of optical density of lutein and zeaxanthin in retinas of older women in the Carotenoids in Age-Related Eye Disease Study, an ancillary study of the Women's Health Initiative. Am J Clin Nutr. 2006 Nov;84(5):1107-22. doi: 10.1093/ajcn/84.5.1107. PMID: 17093164.

166. Mares-Perlman JA, Brady WE, Klein BE, Klein R, Haus GJ, Palta M, Ritter LL, Shoff SM. Diet and nuclear lens opacities. Am J Epidemiol. 1995 Feb 15;141(4):322-34. doi: 10.1093/aje/141.4.322. PMID: 7840110.

167. Martel JL, Kerndt CC, Doshi H, et al. Vitamin B1 (Thiamine) [Updated 2021 Oct 16]. In: StatPearls [Internet]. Treasure Island (FL): StatPearls Publishing; 2022 Jan-. Available from: https://www.ncbi.nlm.nih.gov/books/NBK482360/.

168. Martí N, Mena P, Cánovas JA, Micol V, Saura D. Vitamin C and the role of citrus juices as functional food. Nat Prod Commun. 2009 May;4(5):677-700. PMID: 19445318.

169. Martín R, Miquel S, Ulmer J, Kechaou N, Langella P, Bermúdez-Humarán LG. Role of commensal and probiotic bacteria in human health: a focus on inflammatory bowel disease. Microb Cell Fact. 2013 Jul 23;12:71. doi: 10.1186/1475-2859-12-71. PMID: 23876056; PMCID: PMC3726476.

170. Matsufuji, H., Ishikawa, K., Nunomura, O., Chino, M. and Takeda, M. (2007), Anti-oxidant content of different coloured sweet peppers, white, green, yellow, orange and red (Capsicum annuum L.). International Journal of Food Science & Technology, 42: 1482-1488. https://doi.org/10.1111/j.1365-2621.2006.01368.x

171. Maurer NE, Hatta-Sakoda B, Pascual-Chagman G, Rodriguez-Saona LE. Characterization and authentication of a novel vegetable source of omega-3 fatty acids, sacha inchi (Plukenetia volubilis L.) oil. Food Chem. 2012 Sep 15;134(2):1173-80. doi: 10.1016/j.foodchem.2012.02.143. Epub 2012 Mar 3. PMID: 23107745.

172. McDermott JH. Antioxidant nutrients: current dietary recommendations and research update. J Am Pharm Assoc (Wash). 2000 Nov-Dec;40(6):785-99. doi: 10.1016/s1086-5802(16)31126-3. PMID: 11111359.

173. McKay TB, Karamichos D. Quercetin and the ocular surface: What we know and where we are going. Exp Biol Med (Maywood). 2017 Mar;242(6):565-572. doi: 10.1177/1535370216685187. Epub 2017 Jan 5. PMID: 28056553; PMCID: PMC5685256.

174. Merle BM, Silver RE, Rosner B, Seddon JM. Adherence to a Mediterranean diet, genetic susceptibility, and progression to advanced macular degeneration: a prospective cohort study. Am J Clin Nutr. 2015 Nov;102(5):1196-206. doi: 10.3945/ajcn.115.111047. Epub 2015 Oct 21. PMID: 26490493; PMCID: PMC4625588.

175. Merle BM, Silver RE, Rosner B, Seddon JM. Dietary folate, B vitamins, genetic susceptibility and progression to advanced nonexudative age-related macular degeneration with geographic atrophy: a prospective cohort study. Am J Clin Nutr. 2016 Apr;103(4):1135-44. doi: 10.3945/ajcn.115.117606. PMID: 26961928; PMCID: PMC4807698.

176. Merle BM, Silver RE, Rosner B, Seddon JM. Dietary folate, B vitamins, genetic susceptibility and progression to advanced nonexudative age-related macular degeneration with geographic atrophy: a prospective cohort study. Am J Clin Nutr. 2016 Apr;103(4):1135-44. doi: 10.3945/ajcn.115.117606. PMID: 26961928; PMCID: PMC4807698.

177. Merle BMJ, Silver RE, Rosner B, Seddon JM. Associations Between Vitamin D Intake and Progression to Incident Advanced Age-Related Macular Degeneration. Invest Ophthalmol Vis Sci. 2017 Sep 1;58(11):4569-4578. doi: 10.1167/iovs.17-21673. PMID: 28892825; PMCID: PMC5595226.

178. Miljanović B, Trivedi KA, Dana MR, Gilbard JP, Buring JE, Schaumberg DA. Relation between dietary n-3 and n-6 fatty acids and clinically diagnosed dry eye syndrome in women. Am J Clin Nutr. 2005 Oct;82(4):887-93. doi: 10.1093/ajcn/82.4.887. PMID: 16210721; PMCID: PMC1360504.

179. Millen AE, Meyers KJ, Liu Z, Engelman CD, Wallace RB, LeBlanc ES, Tinker LF, Iyengar SK, Robinson JG, Sarto GE, Mares JA. Association between vitamin D status and age-related macular degeneration by genetic risk. JAMA Ophthalmol. 2015 Oct;133(10):1171-9. doi: 10.1001/jamaophthalmol.2015.2715. PMID: 26312598; PMCID: PMC4841267.

180. Moeller SM, Parekh N, Tinker L, Ritenbaugh C, Blodi B, Wallace RB, Mares JA; CAREDS Research Study Group. Associations between intermediate age-related macular degeneration and lutein and zeaxanthin in the Carotenoids in Age-related Eye Disease Study (CAREDS): ancillary study of the Women's Health Initiative. Arch Ophthalmol. 2006 Aug;124(8):1151-62. doi: 10.1001/archopht.124.8.1151. PMID: 16908818.

181. Moeller SM, Voland R, Tinker L, Blodi BA, Klein ML, Gehrs KM, Johnson EJ, Snodderly DM, Wallace RB, Chappell RJ, Parekh N, Ritenbaugh C, Mares JA; CAREDS Study Group; Women's Health Initiative. Associations between age-related nuclear cataract and lutein and zeaxanthin in the diet and serum in the Carotenoids in the Age-Related Eye Disease Study, an Ancillary Study of the Women's Health Initiative. Arch Ophthalmol. 2008 Mar;126(3):354-64. doi: 10.1001/archopht.126.3.354. PMID: 18332316; PMCID: PMC2562026.

182. Moeller SM, Taylor A, Tucker KL, McCullough ML, Chylack LT Jr, Hankinson SE, Willett WC, Jacques PF. Overall adherence to the dietary guidelines for Americans is associated with reduced prevalence of early age-related nuclear lens opacities in women. J Nutr. 2004 Jul;134(7):1812-9. doi: 10.1093/jn/134.7.1812. PMID: 15226474.

183. Moon J, Yoon CH, Choi SH, Kim MK. Can Gut Microbiota Affect Dry Eye Syndrome? Int J Mol Sci. 2020 Nov 10;21(22):8443. doi: 10.3390/ijms21228443. PMID: 33182758; PMCID: PMC7697210.

184. Moriya C, Hosoya T, Agawa S, Sugiyama Y, Kozone I, Shin-Ya K, Terahara N, Kumazawa S. New acylated anthocyanins from purple yam and their antioxidant activity. Biosci Biotechnol Biochem. 2015;79(9):1484-92. doi: 10.1080/09168451.2015.1027652. Epub 2015 Apr 7. PMID: 25848974.

185. Mozaffarieh M, Grieshaber MC, Orgül S, Flammer J. The potential value of natural antioxidative treatment in glaucoma. Surv Ophthalmol. 2008 Sep-Oct;53(5):479-505. doi: 10.1016/j.survophthal.2008.06.006. PMID: 18929760.

186. Napolitano P, Filippelli M, Davinelli S, Bartollino S, dell'Omo R, Costagliola C. Influence of gut microbiota on eye diseases: an overview. Ann Med. 2021 Dec;53(1):750-761. doi: 10.1080/07853890.2021.1925150. PMID: 34042554; PMCID: PMC8168766.

187. National Institutes for Health. Vitamin C- Fact Sheet for Professionals. Available at: https://ods.od.nih.gov/factsheets/VitaminC-HealthProfessional/. Accessed 6-2-2022.

188. National Institutes for Health. Probiotics - Fact Sheet for Professionals. Available at: https://ods.od.nih.gov/factsheets/Probiotics-HealthProfessional/. Accessed December 5, 2022.

189. National Institutes for Health, National Cancer Institute. Cruciferous Vegetables and Cancer Prevention. Available at: https://www.cancer.gov/about-cancer/causes-prevention/risk/diet/cruciferous-vegetables-fact-sheet. Accessed July 7, 2022.

190. Nebbioso M, Franzone F, Greco A, Gharbiya M, Bonfiglio V, Polimeni A. Recent Advances and Disputes About Curcumin in Retinal Diseases. Clin Ophthalmol. 2021 Jun 18;15:2553-2571. doi: 10.2147/OPTH.S306706. PMID: 34177257; PMCID: PMC8219301.

191. Nomi Y, Iwasaki-Kurashige K, Matsumoto H. Therapeutic Effects of Anthocyanins for Vision and Eye Health. Molecules. 2019 Sep 11;24(18):3311. doi: 10.3390/molecules24183311. PMID: 31514422; PMCID: PMC6767261.

192. Nourish by WedMD. Health Benefits of Rosemary. Available at: https://www.webmd.com/diet/health-benefits-rosemary. Accessed June 15, 2022.

193. NutritionData. Nuts, almonds [Includes USDA commodity food A256, A264] Nutrition Facts & Calories. Available at: https://nutritiondata.self.com/facts/nut-and-seed-products/3085/2. Accessed October 2, 2022.

194. Obidiegwu JE, Lyons JB, Chilaka CA. The Dioscorea Genus (Yam)-An Appraisal of Nutritional and Therapeutic Potentials. Foods. 2020 Sep 16;9(9):1304. doi: 10.3390/foods9091304. PMID: 32947880; PMCID: PMC7555206.

195. Oguido APMT, Hohmann MSN, Pinho-Ribeiro FA, Crespigio J, Domiciano TP, Verri WA Jr, Casella AMB. Naringenin Eye Drops Inhibit Corneal Neovascularization by Anti-Inflammatory and Antioxidant Mechanisms. Invest Ophthalmol Vis Sci. 2017 Nov 1;58(13):5764-5776. doi: 10.1167/iovs.16-19702. PMID: 29117277.

196. Olmedilla-Alonso B, Rodríguez-Rodríguez E, Beltrán-de-Miguel B, Sánchez-Prieto M, Estévez-Santiago R. Changes in Lutein Status Markers (Serum and Faecal Concentrations, Macular Pigment) in Response to a Lutein-Rich Fruit or Vegetable (Three Pieces/Day) Dietary Intervention in Normolipemic Subjects. Nutrients. 2021 Oct 15;13(10):3614. doi: 10.3390/nu13103614. PMID: 34684614; PMCID: PMC8538254.

197. Ooe E, Ogawa K, Horiuchi T, Tada H, Murase H, Tsuruma K, Shimazawa M, Hara H. Analysis and characterization of anthocyanins and carotenoids in Japanese blue tomato. Biosci Biotechnol Biochem. 2016;80(2):341-9. doi: 10.1080/09168451.2015.1091715. Epub 2015 Oct 7. PMID: 26443075.

198. Organisciak DT, Darrow RM, Rapp CM, Smuts JP, Armstrong DW, Lang JC. Prevention of retinal light damage by zinc oxide combined with rosemary extract. Mol Vis. 2013 Jun 27;19:1433-45. PMID: 23825923; PMCID: PMC3695758.

199. Pagliarini S, Moramarco A, Wormald RP, Piguet B, Carresi C, Balacco-Gabrieli C, Sehmi KS, Bird AC. Age-related macular disease in rural southern Italy. Arch Ophthalmol. 1997 May;115(5):616-22. doi: 10.1001/archopht.1997.01100150618007. PMID: 9152129.

200. Parekh N, Voland RP, Moeller SM, Blodi BA, Ritenbaugh C, Chappell RJ, Wallace RB, Mares JA; CAREDS Research Study Group. Association between dietary fat intake and age-related macular degeneration in the Carotenoids in Age-Related Eye Disease Study (CAREDS): an ancillary study of the Women's Health Initiative. Arch Ophthalmol. 2009 Nov;127(11):1483-93. doi: 10.1001/archophthalmol.2009.130. PMID: 19901214; PMCID: PMC3144752.

201. Parekh N, Chappell RJ, Millen AE, Albert DM, Mares JA. Association between vitamin D and age-related macular degeneration in the Third National Health and Nutrition Examination Survey, 1988 through 1994. Arch Ophthalmol. 2007 May;125(5):661-9. doi: 10.1001/archopht.125.5.661. PMID: 17502506.

202. Park CM, Cho CW, Song YS. TOP 1 and 2, polysaccharides from Taraxacum officinale, inhibit NFκB-mediated inflammation and accelerate Nrf2-induced antioxidative potential through the modulation of PI3K-Akt signaling pathway in RAW 264.7 cells. Food Chem Toxicol. 2014 Apr;66:56-64. doi: 10.1016/j.fct.2014.01.019. Epub 2014 Jan 18. PMID: 24447978.

203. Pellegrini M, Senni C, Bernabei F, Cicero AFG, Vagge A, Maestri A, Scorcia V, Giannaccare G. The Role of Nutrition and Nutritional Supplements in Ocular Surface Diseases. Nutrients. 2020 Mar 30;12(4):952. doi: 10.3390/nu12040952. PMID: 32235501; PMCID: PMC7230622.

204. Piccardi M, Marangoni D, Minnella AM, Savastano MC, Valentini P, Ambrosio L, Capoluongo E, Maccarone R, Bisti S, Falsini B. A longitudinal follow-up study of saffron supplementation in early age-related macular degeneration: sustained benefits to central retinal function. Evid Based Complement Alternat Med. 2012;2012:429124. doi: 10.1155/2012/429124. Epub 2012 Jul 18. PMID: 22852021; PMCID: PMC3407634.

205. Ponder A, Kulik K, Hallmann E. Occurrence and Determination of Carotenoids and Polyphenols in Different Paprika Powders from Organic and Conventional Production. Molecules. 2021 May 17;26(10):2980. doi: 10.3390/molecules26102980. PMID: 34067891; PMCID: PMC8156602.

206. Qureshi AI, Suri FK, Ahmed S, Nasar A, Divani AA, Kirmani JF. Regular egg consumption does not increase the risk of stroke and cardiovascular diseases. Med Sci Monit. 2007 Jan;13(1):CR1-8. Epub 2006 Dec 18. PMID: 17179903.

207. Radomska-Leśniewska DM, Osiecka-Iwan A, Hyc A, Góźdź A, Dąbrowska AM, Skopiński P. Therapeutic potential of curcumin in eye diseases. Cent Eur J Immunol. 2019;44(2):181-189. doi: 10.5114/ceji.2019.87070. Epub 2019 Jul 30. PMID: 31530988; PMCID: PMC6745545.

208. Rakhshan R, Atashi HA, Hoseinian M, Jafari A, Haghighi A, Ziyadloo F, Razizadeh N, Ghasemian H, Nia MMK, Sefidi AB, Arani HZ. The Synergistic Cytotoxic and Apoptotic Effect of Resveratrol and Naringenin on Y79 Retinoblastoma Cell Line. Anticancer Agents Med Chem. 2021 Oct 28;21(16):2243-2249. doi: 10.2174/1871520621666210112121051. PMID: 33438556.

209. Raman R, Vaghefi E, Braakhuis AJ. Food components and ocular pathophysiology: a critical appraisal of the role of oxidative mechanisms. Asia Pac J Clin Nutr. 2017;26(4):572-585. doi: 10.6133/apjcn.082016.01. PMID: 28582804.

210. Ramdas WD. The relation between dietary intake and glaucoma: a systematic review. Acta Ophthalmol. 2018 Sep;96(6):550-556. doi: 10.1111/aos.13662. Epub 2018 Feb 20. PMID: 29461678.

211. Rao P, Millen AE, Meyers KJ, Liu Z, Voland R, Sondel S, Tinker L, Wallace RB, Blodi BA, Binkley N, Sarto G, Robinson J, LeBlanc E, Mares JA. The Relationship Between Serum 25-Hydroxyvitamin D Levels and Nuclear Cataract in the Carotenoid Age-Related Eye Study (CAREDS), an Ancillary Study of the Women's Health Initiative. Invest Ophthalmol Vis Sci. 2015 Jul;56(8):4221-30. doi: 10.1167/iovs.15-16835. PMID: 26132781; PMCID: PMC4495813.

212. Reddy VN, Giblin FJ, Lin LR, Chakrapani B. The effect of aqueous humor ascorbate on ultraviolet-B-induced DNA damage in lens epithelium. Invest Ophthalmol Vis Sci. 1998 Feb;39(2):344-50. PMID: 9477992.

213. Reynolds R, Rosner B, Seddon JM. Dietary omega-3 fatty acids, other fat intake, genetic susceptibility, and progression to incident geographic atrophy. Ophthalmology. 2013 May;120(5):1020-8. doi: 10.1016/j.ophtha.2012.10.020. Epub 2013 Mar 5. PMID: 23481534; PMCID: PMC3758110.

214. Richer S, Stiles W, Statkute L, Pulido J, Frankowski J, Rudy D, Pei K, Tsipursky M, Nyland J. Double-masked, placebo-controlled, randomized trial of lutein and antioxidant supplementation in the intervention of atrophic age-related macular degeneration: the Veterans LAST study (Lutein Antioxidant Supplementation Trial). Optometry. 2004 Apr;75(4):216-30. doi: 10.1016/s1529-1839(04)70049-4. PMID: 15117055.

215. Richer SP, Stiles W, Graham-Hoffman K, Levin M, Ruskin D, Wrobel J, Park DW, Thomas C. Randomized, double-blind, placebo-controlled study of zeaxanthin and visual function in patients with atrophic age-related macular degeneration: the Zeaxanthin and Visual Function Study (ZVF) FDA IND #78, 973. Optometry. 2011 Nov;82(11):667-680.e6. doi: 10.1016/j.optm.2011.08.008. PMID: 22027699.

216. Rinninella E, Mele MC, Merendino N, Cintoni M, Anselmi G, Caporossi A, Gasbarrini A, Minnella AM. The Role of Diet, Micronutrients and the Gut Microbiota in Age-Related Macular Degeneration: New Perspectives from the Gut-Retina Axis. Nutrients. 2018 Nov 5;10(11):1677. doi: 10.3390/nu10111677. PMID: 30400586; PMCID: PMC6267253.

217. Roh M, Shin HJ, Laíns I, Providência J, Caseiro-Alves M, Barreto P, Vavvas DG, Miller JB, Kim IK, Gaziano JM, Liang L, Silva R, Miller JW, Husain D. Higher Intake of Polyunsaturated Fatty Acid and Monounsaturated Fatty Acid is Inversely Associated With AMD. Invest Ophthalmol Vis Sci. 2020 Feb 7;61(2):20. doi: 10.1167/iovs.61.2.20. PMID: 32058563; PMCID: PMC7326508.

218. Saiki P, Yoshihara M, Kawano Y, Miyazaki H, Miyazaki K. Anti-Inflammatory Effects of Heliangin from Jerusalem Artichoke (Helianthus tuberosus) Leaves Might Prevent Atherosclerosis. Biomolecules. 2022 Jan 6;12(1):91. doi: 10.3390/biom12010091. PMID: 35053238; PMCID: PMC8774036.

219. Salehi B, Stojanović-Radić Z, Matejić J, Sharifi-Rad M, Anil Kumar NV, Martins N, Sharifi-Rad J. The therapeutic potential of curcumin: A review of clinical trials. Eur J Med Chem. 2019 Feb 1;163:527-545. doi: 10.1016/j.ejmech.2018.12.016. Epub 2018 Dec 7. PMID: 30553144.

220. Sampath C, Sang S, Ahmedna M. In vitro and in vivo inhibition of aldose reductase and advanced glycation end products by phloretin, epigallocatechin 3-gallate and [6]-gingerol. Biomed Pharmacother. 2016 Dec;84:502-513. doi: 10.1016/j.biopha.2016.09.073. Epub 2016 Sep 28. PMID: 27685794.

221. SanGiovanni JP, Chew EY. The role of omega-3 long-chain polyunsaturated fatty acids in health and disease of the retina. Prog Retin Eye Res. 2005 Jan;24(1):87-138. doi: 10.1016/j.preteyeres.2004.06.002. PMID: 15555528.

222. SanGiovanni JP, Agrón E, Clemons TE, Chew EY. Omega-3 long-chain polyunsaturated fatty acid intake inversely associated with 12-year progression to advanced age-related macular degeneration. Arch Ophthalmol. 2009 Jan;127(1):110-2. doi: 10.1001/archophthalmol.2008.518. PMID: 19139352; PMCID: PMC2812062.

223. SanGiovanni JP, Chew EY, Clemons TE, Davis MD, Ferris FL 3rd, Gensler GR, Kurinij N, Lindblad AS, Milton RC, Seddon JM, Sperduto RD; Age-Related Eye Disease Study Research Group. The relationship of dietary lipid intake and age-related macular degeneration in a case-control study: AREDS Report No. 20. Arch Ophthalmol. 2007 May;125(5):671-9. doi: 10.1001/archopht.125.5.671. PMID: 17502507.

224. SanGiovanni JP, Chew EY, Agrón E, Clemons TE, Ferris FL 3rd, Gensler G, Lindblad AS, Milton RC, Seddon JM, Klein R, Sperduto RD; Age-Related Eye Disease Study Research Group. The relationship of dietary omega-3 long-chain polyunsaturated fatty acid intake with incident age-related macular degeneration: AREDS report no. 23. Arch Ophthalmol. 2008 Sep;126(9):1274-9. doi: 10.1001/archopht.126.9.1274. PMID: 18779490; PMCID: PMC2812063.

225. Sangiovanni JP, Agrón E, Meleth AD, Reed GF, Sperduto RD, Clemons TE, Chew EY; Age-Related Eye Disease Study Research Group. {omega}-3 Long-chain polyunsaturated fatty acid intake and 12-y incidence of neovascular age-related macular degeneration and central geographic atrophy: AREDS report 30, a prospective cohort study from the Age-Related Eye Disease Study. Am J Clin Nutr. 2009 Dec;90(6):1601-7. doi: 10.3945/ajcn.2009.27594. Epub 2009 Oct 7. PMID: 19812176; PMCID: PMC2777471.

226. Satija A, Hu FB. Plant-based diets and cardiovascular health. Trends Cardiovasc Med. 2018 Oct;28(7):437-441. doi: 10.1016/j.tcm.2018.02.004. Epub 2018 Feb 13. PMID: 29496410; PMCID: PMC6089671.

227. Sawicka B, Skiba D, Pszczółkowski P, Aslan I, Sharifi-Rad J, Krochmal-Marczak B. Jerusalem artichoke (Helianthus tuberosus L.) as a medicinal plant and its natural products. Cell Mol Biol (Noisy-le-grand). 2020 Jun 25;66(4):160-177. PMID: 32583794.

228. Schrier SA, Falk MJ. Mitochondrial disorders and the eye. Curr Opin Ophthalmol. 2011 Sep;22(5):325-31. doi: 10.1097/ICU.0b013e328349419d. PMID: 21730846; PMCID: PMC3652603.

229. ScienceBased Health. ScienceBased Health Response to the DREAM Study on Fish Oil for Dry Eye. Available at https://www.sciencebasedhealth.com/Response-to-the-DREAM-Study-on-Fish-Oil-for-Dry-Eye-W702.aspx. Accessed 9-16-2022.

230. Seddon JM. Multivitamin-multimineral supplements and eye disease: age-related macular degeneration and cataract. Am J Clin Nutr. 2007 Jan;85(1):304S-307S. doi: 10.1093/ajcn/85.1.304S. PMID: 17209215.

231. Seddon JM. Macular Degeneration Epidemiology: Nature-Nurture, Lifestyle Factors, Genetic Risk, and Gene-Environment Interactions - The Weisenfeld Award Lecture. Invest Ophthalmol Vis Sci. 2017 Dec 1;58(14):6513-6528. doi: 10.1167/iovs.17-23544. PMID: 29288272; PMCID: PMC5749242.

232. Seddon JM, Widjajahakim R, Rosner B. Rare and Common Genetic Variants, Smoking, and Body Mass Index: Progression and Earlier Age of Developing Advanced Age-Related Macular Degeneration. Invest Ophthalmol Vis Sci. 2020 Dec 1;61(14):32. doi: 10.1167/iovs.61.14.32. PMID: 33369641; PMCID: PMC7774056.

233. Seddon JM, Christen WG, Manson JE, LaMotte FS, Glynn RJ, Buring JE, Hennekens CH. The use of vitamin supplements and the risk of cataract among US male physicians. Am J Public Health. 1994 May;84(5):788-92. doi: 10.2105/ajph.84.5.788. PMID: 8179050; PMCID: PMC1615060.

234. Seddon JM, Rosner B, Sperduto RD, Yannuzzi L, Haller JA, Blair NP, Willett W. Dietary fat and risk for advanced age-related macular degeneration. Arch Ophthalmol. 2001 Aug;119(8):1191-9. doi: 10.1001/archopht.119.8.1191. PMID: 11483088.

235. Seddon JM, Gensler G, Klein ML, Milton RC. C-reactive protein and homocysteine are associated with dietary and behavioral risk factors for age-related macular degeneration. Nutrition. 2006 Apr;22(4):441-3. doi: 10.1016/j.nut.2005.12.004. PMID: 16530626.

236. Seddon JM, Cote J, Davis N, Rosner B. Progression of age-related macular degeneration: association with body mass index, waist circumference, and waist-hip ratio. Arch Ophthalmol. 2003 Jun;121(6):785-92. doi: 10.1001/archopht.121.6.785. PMID: 12796248

237. Seddon JM, George S, Rosner B. Cigarette smoking, fish consumption, omega-3 fatty acid intake, and associations with age-related macular degeneration: the US Twin Study of Age-Related Macular Degeneration. Arch Ophthalmol. 2006 Jul;124(7):995-1001. doi: 10.1001/archopht.124.7.995. PMID: 16832023.

238. Seddon JM, Ajani UA, Sperduto RD, Hiller R, Blair N, Burton TC, Farber MD, Gragoudas ES, Haller J, Miller DT, et al. Dietary carotenoids, vitamins A, C, and E, and advanced age-related macular degeneration. Eye Disease Case-Control Study Group. JAMA. 1994 Nov 9;272(18):1413-20. Erratum in: JAMA 1995 Feb 22;273(8):622. PMID: 7933422.

239. Seddon JM, Reynolds R, Shah HR, Rosner B. Smoking, dietary betaine, methionine, and vitamin D in monozygotic twins with discordant macular degeneration: epigenetic implications. Ophthalmology. 2011 Jul;118(7):1386-94. doi: 10.1016/j.ophtha.2010.12.020. Epub 2011 May 28. PMID: 21620475; PMCID: PMC3711586.

240. Sherwin JC, Kokavec J, Thornton SN. Hydration, fluid regulation and the eye: in health and disease. Clin Exp Ophthalmol. 2015 Nov;43(8):749-64. doi: 10.1111/ceo.12546. Epub 2015 Jun 19. PMID: 25950246.

241. Shivaji S. Connect between gut microbiome and diseases of the human eye. J Biosci. 2019 Oct;44(5):110. PMID: 31719219.

242. Shoda H, Yanai R, Yoshimura T, Nagai T, Kimura K, Sobrin L, Connor KM, Sakoda Y, Tamada K, Ikeda T, Sonoda KH. Dietary Omega-3 Fatty Acids Suppress Experimental Autoimmune Uveitis in Association with Inhibition of Th1 and Th17 Cell Function. PLoS One. 2015 Sep 22;10(9):e0138241. doi: 10.1371/journal.pone.0138241. PMID: 26393358; PMCID: PMC4578775.

243. Sinclair AJ, Guo XF, Abedin L. Dietary Alpha-Linolenic Acid Supports High Retinal DHA Levels. Nutrients. 2022 Jan 12;14(2):301. doi: 10.3390/nu14020301. PMID: 35057481; PMCID: PMC8779487.

244. Song H, Wang YH, Zhou HY, Cui KM. Sulforaphane alleviates LPS-induced inflammatory injury in ARPE-19 cells by repressing the PWRN2/NF-kB pathway. Immunopharmacol Immunotoxicol. 2022 Jun 29:1-9. doi: 10.1080/08923973.2022.2090954. Epub ahead of print. PMID: 35766158.

245. Song M, Fung TT, Hu FB, Willett WC, Longo VD, Chan AT, Giovannucci EL. Association of Animal and Plant Protein Intake With All-Cause and Cause-Specific Mortality. JAMA Intern Med. 2016 Oct 1;176(10):1453-1463. doi: 10.1001/jamainternmed.2016.4182. Erratum in: JAMA Intern Med. 2016 Nov 1;176(11):1728. PMID: 27479196; PMCID: PMC5048552.

246. Sperduto RD, Hu TS, Milton RC, Zhao JL, Everett DF, Cheng QF, Blot WJ, Bing L, Taylor PR, Li JY, et al. The Linxian cataract studies. Two nutrition intervention trials. Arch Ophthalmol. 1993 Sep;111(9):1246-53. doi: 10.1001/archopht.1993.01090090098027. PMID: 8363468.

247. Srivichai S, Hongsprabhas P. Profiling Anthocyanins in Thai Purple Yams (Dioscorea alata L.). Int J Food Sci. 2020 Jul 9;2020:1594291. doi: 10.1155/2020/1594291. PMID: 32695807; PMCID: PMC7368940.

248. Sun T, Xu Z, Wu CT, Janes M, Prinyawiwatkul W, No HK. Antioxidant activities of different colored sweet bell peppers (Capsicum annuum L.). J Food Sci. 2007 Mar;72(2):S98-102. doi: 10.1111/j.1750-3841.2006.00245.x. PMID: 17995862.

249. Tan AG, Mitchell P, Flood VM, Burlutsky G, Rochtchina E, Cumming RG, Wang JJ. Antioxidant nutrient intake and the long-term incidence of age-related cataract: the Blue Mountains Eye Study. Am J Clin Nutr. 2008 Jun;87(6):1899-905. doi: 10.1093/ajcn/87.6.1899. PMID: 18541583.

250. Tan JS, Wang JJ, Flood V, Mitchell P. Dietary fatty acids and the 10-year incidence of age-related macular degeneration: the Blue Mountains Eye Study. Arch Ophthalmol. 2009 May;127(5):656-65. doi: 10.1001/archophthalmol.2009.76. PMID: 19433717.

251. Tan JS, Wang JJ, Flood V, Rochtchina E, Smith W, Mitchell P. Dietary antioxidants and the long-term incidence of age-related macular degeneration: the Blue Mountains Eye Study. Ophthalmology. 2008 Feb;115(2):334-41. doi: 10.1016/j.ophtha.2007.03.083. Epub 2007 Jul 30. PMID: 17664009.

252. Tang D, Mitchell P, Flood V, Kifley A, Hayes A, Liew G, Gopinath B. Dietary intervention in patients with age-related macular degeneration: protocol for a randomised controlled trial. BMJ Open. 2019 Feb 19;9(2):e024774. doi: 10.1136/bmjopen-2018-024774. PMID: 30782917; PMCID: PMC6377551.

253. Tang D, Mitchell P, Liew G, Burlutsky G, Flood V, Gopinath B. Evaluation of a Novel Tool for Screening Inadequate Food Intake in Age-Related Macular Degeneration Patients. Nutrients. 2019 Dec 12;11(12):3031. doi: 10.3390/nu11123031. PMID: 31842257; PMCID: PMC6949902.

254. Tavani A, Negri E, La Vecchia C. Food and nutrient intake and risk of cataract. Ann Epidemiol. 1996 Jan;6(1):41-6. doi: 10.1016/1047-2797(95)00099-2. PMID: 8680624.

255. Taylor A, Jacques PF, Chylack LT Jr, Hankinson SE, Khu PM, Rogers G, Friend J, Tung W, Wolfe JK, Padhye N, Willett WC. Long-term intake of vitamins and carotenoids and odds of early age-related cortical and posterior subcapsular lens opacities. Am J Clin Nutr. 2002 Mar;75(3):540-9. doi: 10.1093/ajcn/75.3.540. PMID: 11864861.

256. Thompson SV, Bailey MA, Taylor AM, Kaczmarek JL, Mysonhimer AR, Edwards CG, Reeser GE, Burd NA, Khan NA, Holscher HD. Avocado Consumption Alters Gastrointestinal Bacteria Abundance and Microbial Metabolite Concentrations among Adults with Overweight or Obesity: A Randomized Controlled Trial. J Nutr. 2021 Apr 8;151(4):753-762. doi: 10.1093/jn/nxaa219. PMID: 32805028; PMCID: PMC8030699.

257. Tomany SC, Cruickshanks KJ, Klein R, Klein BE, Knudtson MD. Sunlight and the 10-year incidence of age-related maculopathy: the Beaver Dam Eye Study. Arch Ophthalmol. 2004 May;122(5):750-7. doi: 10.1001/archopht.122.5.750. Erratum in: Arch Ophthalmol. 2005 Mar;123(3):362. PMID: 15136324.

258. Totsch SK, Meir RY, Quinn TL, Lopez SA, Gower BA, Sorge RE. Effects of a Standard American Diet and an anti-inflammatory diet in male and female mice. Eur J Pain. 2018 Aug;22(7):1203-1213. doi: 10.1002/ejp.1207. Epub 2018 Mar 2. PMID: 29436058.

259. Tosini G, Ferguson I, Tsubota K. Effects of blue light on the circadian system and eye physiology. Mol Vis. 2016 Jan 24;22:61-72. PMID: 26900325; PMCID: PMC4734149.

260. Townend BS, Townend ME, Flood V, Burlutsky G, Rochtchina E, Wang JJ, Mitchell P. Dietary macronutrient intake and five-year incident cataract: the blue mountains eye study. Am J Ophthalmol. 2007 Jun;143(6):932-939. doi: 10.1016/j.ajo.2007.03.006. Epub 2007 Apr 24. PMID: 17459316.

261. Truswell AS, Mitchell P. Nutrients and degenerative eye diseases. Asia Pac J Clin Nutr. 1993 Nov;2 Suppl 1:47-50. PMID: 24398183.

262. Ullah R, Nadeem M, Khalique A, Imran M, Mehmood S, Javid A, Hussain J. Nutritional and therapeutic perspectives of Chia (Salvia hispanica L.): a review. J Food Sci Technol. 2016 Apr;53(4):1750-8. doi: 10.1007/s13197-015-1967-0. Epub 2015 Oct 1. PMID: 27413203; PMCID: PMC4926888.

263. United States Department of Agriculture, Agricultural Research Service. USDA food composition databases. Available at: https://www.ars.usda.gov/arsuserfiles/80400525/data/hg72/hg72_2002.pdf. Accessed June 1, 2022.

264. United States Department of Agriculture, Agricultural Research Service. USDA food composition. Available at: https://www.nal.usda.gov/human-nutrition-and-food-safety/food-composition. Accessed June 1, 2022.'

265. United States Department of Agriculture, Agricultural Research Service. FoodData Central. Available at: https://fdc.nal.usda.gov/fdc-app.html. Accessed June 1, 2022.

266. United States Department of Agriculture, Agricultural Research Service. FoodData Central. Available at: https://fdc.nal.usda.gov/fdc-app.html#/food-details/171705/nutrients. Accessed June 1, 2022.

267. United States Department of Agriculture, Agricultural Research Service. FoodData Central. Available at: https://fdc.nal.usda.gov/fdc-app.html#/food-details/171719/nutrients. Accessed June 15, 2022.

268. United States Department of Agriculture, Agricultural Research Service. FoodData Central. Available at: https://fdc.nal.usda.gov/fdc-app.html#/food-details/170554/nutrients. Accessed June 15, 2022.

269. United States Department of Agriculture, Agricultural Research Service. FoodData Central. Available at: https://fdc.nal.usda.gov/fdc-app.html#/food-details/169226/nutrients. Accessed June 3, 2022.

270. United States Department of Agriculture, Agricultural Research Service. FoodData Central. Available at: https://fdc.nal.usda.gov/fdc-app.html#/food-details/169236/nutrients. Accessed June 3, 2022.

271. United States Department of Agriculture, Agricultural Research Service. FoodData Central. Available at: https://fdc.nal.usda.gov/fdc-app.html#/food-details/170073/nutrients. Accessed June 3, 2022.

272. United States Department of Agriculture, Agricultural Research Service. FoodData Central. Available at: https://fdc.nal.usda.gov/fdc-app.html#/food-details/327357/nutrients. Accessed June 30, 2022.

273. United States Department of Agriculture, Agricultural Research Service. FoodData Central. Available at: https://fdc.nal.usda.gov/fdc-app.html#/food-details/1102667/nutrients. Accessed June 3, 2022.

274. United States Department of Agriculture, Agricultural Research Service. *FoodData Central*. Available at: https://fdc.nal.usda.gov/fdc-app.html#/food-details/171329/nutrients. Accessed June 14, 2022.

275. United States Department of Agriculture, Agricultural Research Service. *FoodData Central*. Available at: https://fdc.nal.usda.gov/fdc-app.html#/food-details/170416/nutrients. Accessed June 14, 2022.

276. United States Department of Agriculture, Agricultural Research Service. *FoodData Central*. Available at: https://fdc.nal.usda.gov/fdc-app.html#/food-details/170184/nutrients. Accessed June 14, 2022.

277. United States Department of Agriculture, Agricultural Research Service. *FoodData Central*. Available at: https://fdc.nal.usda.gov/fdc-app.html#/food-details/169134/nutrients. Accessed June 14, 2022.

278. United States Department of Agriculture, Agricultural Research Service. FoodData Central. Available at: https://fdc.nal.usda.gov/fdc-app.html#/food-details/168917/nutrients. Accessed June 15, 2022.

279. United States Department of Agriculture, Agricultural Research Service. FoodData Central. Available at: https://fdc.nal.usda.gov/fdc-app.html#/food-details/170495/nutrients. Accessed June 15, 2022.

280. United States Department of Agriculture, Agricultural Research Service. FoodData Central. Available at: https://fdc.nal.usda.gov/fdc-app.html#/food-details/1999634/nutrients. Accessed June 15, 2022.

281. United States Department of Agriculture, Agricultural Research Service. FoodData Central. Available at: https://fdc.nal.usda.gov/fdc-app.html#/food-details/172231/nutrients. Accessed June 15, 2022.

282. United States Department of Agriculture, Agricultural Research Service. FoodData Central. Available at: https://fdc.nal.usda.gov/fdc-app.html#/food-details/167765/nutrients. Accessed June 29, 2022.

283. United States Department of Agriculture, Agricultural Research Service. FoodData Central. Available at: https://fdc.nal.usda.gov/fdc-app.html#/food-details/170072/nutrients. Accessed June 30, 2022.

284. United States Department of Agriculture, Agricultural Research Service. FoodData Central. Available at: https://fdc.nal.usda.gov/fdc-app.html#/food-details/168565/nutrients. Accessed June 30, 2022.

285. United States Department of Agriculture, Agricultural Research Service. FoodData Central. Available at: https://fdc.nal.usda.gov/fdc-app.html#/food-details/2111517/nutrients. Accessed June 30, 2022.

286. United States Department of Agriculture, MyPlate. Available at: https://www.myplate.gov/eat-healthy/vegetables. Accessed August 3, 2022.

287. Valero-Vello M, Peris-Martínez C, García-Medina JJ, Sanz-González SM, Ramírez AI, Fernández-Albarral JA, Galarreta-Mira D, Zanón-Moreno V, Casaroli-Marano RP, Pinazo-Duran MD. Searching for the Antioxidant, Anti-Inflammatory, and Neuroprotective Potential of Natural Food and Nutritional Supplements for Ocular Health in the Mediterranean Population. Foods. 2021 May 28;10(6):1231. doi: 10.3390/foods10061231. PMID: 34071459; PMCID: PMC8229954.

288. van Leeuwen R, Boekhoorn S, Vingerling JR, Witteman JC, Klaver CC, Hofman A, de Jong PT. Dietary intake of antioxidants and risk of age-related macular degeneration. JAMA. 2005 Dec 28;294(24):3101-7. doi: 10.1001/jama.294.24.3101. PMID: 16380590.

289. Vavvas DG, Small KW, Awh CC, Zanke BW, Tibshirani RJ, Kustra R. CFH and ARMS2 genetic risk determines progression to neovascular age-related macular degeneration after antioxidant and zinc supplementation. Proc Natl Acad Sci U S A. 2018 Jan 23;115(4):E696-E704. doi: 10.1073/pnas.1718059115. Epub 2018 Jan 8. PMID: 29311295; PMCID: PMC5789949.

290. Vishwanathan R, Schalch W, Johnson EJ. Macular pigment carotenoids in the retina and occipital cortex are related in humans. Nutr Neurosci. 2016;19(3):95-101. doi: 10.1179/1476830514Y.0000000141. Epub 2015 Mar 9. PMID: 25752849.

291. Vučić V, Grabež M, Trchounian A, Arsić A. Composition and Potential Health Benefits of Pomegranate: A Review. Curr Pharm Des. 2019;25(16):1817-1827. doi: 10.2174/1381612825666190708183941. PMID: 31298147.

292. Wallace TC, Slavin M, Frankenfeld CL. Systematic Review of Anthocyanins and Markers of Cardiovascular Disease. Nutrients. 2016 Jan 9;8(1):32. doi: 10.3390/nu8010032. PMID: 26761031; PMCID: PMC4728646.

293. Wang DD, Nguyen LH, Li Y, Yan Y, Ma W, Rinott E, Ivey KL, Shai I, Willett WC, Hu FB, Rimm EB, Stampfer MJ, Chan AT, Huttenhower C. The gut microbiome modulates the protective association between a Mediterranean diet and cardiometabolic disease risk. Nat Med. 2021 Feb;27(2):333-343. doi: 10.1038/s41591-020-01223-3. Epub 2021 Feb 11. PMID: 33574608; PMCID: PMC8186452.

294. Wang L, Tao L, Hao L, Stanley TH, Huang KH, Lambert JD, Kris-Etherton PM. A Moderate-Fat Diet with One Avocado per Day Increases Plasma Antioxidants and Decreases the Oxidation of Small, Dense LDL in Adults with Overweight and Obesity: A Randomized Controlled Trial. J Nutr. 2020 Feb 1;150(2):276-284. doi: 10.1093/jn/nxz231. PMID: 31616932; PMCID: PMC7373821.

295. Wang Y, Huang F, Zhao L, Zhang D, Wang O, Guo X, Lu F, Yang X, Ji B, Deng Q. Protective Effect of Total Flavones from Hippophae rhamnoides L. against Visible Light-Induced Retinal Degeneration in Pigmented Rabbits. J Agric Food Chem. 2016 Jan 13;64(1):161-70. doi: 10.1021/acs.jafc.5b04874. Epub 2015 Dec 23. PMID: 26653970.

296. Weintraub JM, Willett WC, Rosner B, Colditz GA, Seddon JM, Hankinson SE. A prospective study of the relationship between body mass index and cataract extraction among US women and men. Int J Obes Relat Metab Disord. 2002 Dec;26(12):1588-95. doi: 10.1038/sj.ijo.0802158. PMID: 12461675.

297. West S, Vitale S, Hallfrisch J, Muñoz B, Muller D, Bressler S, Bressler NM. Are antioxidants or supplements protective for age-related macular degeneration? Arch Ophthalmol. 1994 Feb;112(2):222-7. doi: 10.1001/archopht.1994.01090140098031. PMID: 8311777.

298. Whitehead AJ, Mares JA, Danis RP. Macular pigment: a review of current knowledge. Arch Ophthalmol. 2006 Jul;124(7):1038-45. doi: 10.1001/archopht.124.7.1038. PMID: 16832030.

299. Widomska J, SanGiovanni JP, Subczynski WK. Why is Zeaxanthin the Most Concentrated Xanthophyll in the Central Fovea? Nutrients. 2020 May 7;12(5):1333. doi: 10.3390/nu12051333. PMID: 32392888; PMCID: PMC7284714.

300. Wien M, Bleich D, Raghuwanshi M, Gould-Forgerite S, Gomes J, Monahan-Couch L, Oda K. Almond consumption and cardiovascular risk factors in adults with prediabetes. J Am Coll Nutr. 2010 Jun;29(3):189-97. doi: 10.1080/07315724.2010.10719833. PMID: 20833991.

301. Wilkinson JT, Fraunfelder FW. Use of herbal medicines and nutritional supplements in ocular disorders: an evidence-based review. Drugs. 2011 Dec 24;71(18):2421-34. doi: 10.2165/11596840-000000000-00000. PMID: 22141385.

302. Willshire C, Bron AJ, Gaffney EA, Pearce EI. Basal Tear Osmolarity as a metric to estimate body hydration and dry eye severity. Prog Retin Eye Res. 2018 May;64:56-64. doi: 10.1016/j.preteyeres.2018.02.001. Epub 2018 Feb 21. PMID: 29476817.

303. Wirngo FE, Lambert MN, Jeppesen PB. The Physiological Effects of Dandelion (Taraxacum Officinale) in Type 2 Diabetes. Rev Diabet Stud. 2016 Summer-Fall;13(2-3):113-131. doi: 10.1900/RDS.2016.13.113. Epub 2016 Aug 10. PMID: 28012278; PMCID: PMC5 553762

304. Wise LA, Rosenberg L, Radin RG, Mattox C, Yang EB, Palmer JR, Seddon JM. A prospective study of diabetes, lifestyle factors, and glaucoma among African-American women. Ann Epidemiol. 2011 Jun;21(6):430-9. doi: 10.1016/j.annepidem.2011.03.006. PMID: 21549278; PMCID: PMC3091261.

305. Wolfe KL, Kang X, He X, Dong M, Zhang Q, Liu RH. Cellular antioxidant activity of common fruits. J Agric Food Chem. 2008 Sep 24;56(18):8418-26. doi: 10.1021/jf801381y. Epub 2008 Aug 30. PMID: 18759450.

306. Wong P, Markey M, Rapp CM, Darrow RM, Ziesel A, Organisciak DT. Enhancing the efficacy of AREDS antioxidants in light-induced retinal degeneration. Mol Vis. 2017 Oct 10;23:718-739. PMID: 29062223; PMCID: PMC5640517.

307. Woodside JV, McGrath AJ, Lyner N, McKinley MC. Carotenoids and health in older people. Maturitas. 2015 Jan;80(1):63-8. doi: 10.1016/j.maturitas.2014.10.012. Epub 2014 Oct 31. PMID: 25466302.

308. Wu J, Cho E, Giovannucci EL, Rosner BA, Sastry SM, Schaumberg DA, Willett WC. Dietary intake of α-linolenic acid and risk of age-related macular degeneration. Am J Clin Nutr. 2017 Jun;105(6):1483-1492. doi: 10.3945/ajcn.116.143453. Epub 2017 May 3. PMID: 28468892; PMCID: PMC5445670.

309. Xue W, Li JJ, Zou Y, Zou B, Wei L. Microbiota and Ocular Diseases. Front Cell Infect Microbiol. 2021 Oct 21;11:759333. doi: 10.3389/fcimb.2021.759333. PMID: 34746029; PMCID: PMC8566696.

310. Yang PM, Wu ZZ, Zhang YQ, Wung BS. Lycopene inhibits ICAM-1 expression and NF-κB activation by Nrf2-regulated cell redox state in human retinal pigment epithelial cells. Life Sci. 2016 Jun 15;155:94-101. doi: 10.1016/j.lfs.2016.05.006. Epub 2016 May 4. PMID: 27155396.

311. Yang Y, Xu C, Chen Y, Liang JJ, Xu Y, Chen SL, Huang S, Yang Q, Cen LP, Pang CP, Sun XH, Ng TK. Green Tea Extract Ameliorates Ischemia-Induced Retinal Ganglion Cell Degeneration in Rats. Oxid Med Cell Longev. 2019 Jul 9;2019:8407206. doi: 10.1155/2019/8407206. PMID: 31379990; PMCID: PMC6652088.

312. Zwart SR, Gregory JF, Zeisel SH, Gibson CR, Mader TH, Kinchen JM, Ueland PM, Ploutz-Snyder R, Heer MA, Smith SM. Genotype, B-vitamin status, and androgens affect spaceflight-induced ophthalmic changes. FASEB J. 2016 Jan;30(1):141-8. doi: 10.1096/fj.15-278457. Epub 2015 Aug 27. PMID: 26316272; PMCID: PMC4684521.

313. Zysset-Burri DC, Morandi S, Herzog EL, Berger LE, Zinkernagel MS. The role of the gut microbiome in eye diseases. Prog Retin Eye Res. 2023 Jan;92:101117. doi: 10.1016/j.preteyeres.2022.101117. Epub 2022 Sep 6. PMID: 36075807.

About the Author

Dr. Rani (Rudrani) Banik is a board-certified ophthalmologist, fellowship-trained neuro-ophthalmologist, and certified functional medicine practitioner.

Dr. Banik offers the best traditional management of ophthalmic disease, combined with an integrative approach. Her treatment protocols promote eye and brain health based on nutrition, botanicals, lifestyle modification, movement, essential oils, and supplements.

Dr. Banik is the founder of EnVision Health, a private practice in New York City. Dr. Banik is an Associate Professor of Ophthalmology at Mount Sinai's Icahn School of Medicine, where she is involved in clinical trials research and teaching. She has authored numerous articles and has presented at national and international meetings. She is a Castle Connolly Top Doctor and New York Magazine Best Doctor.

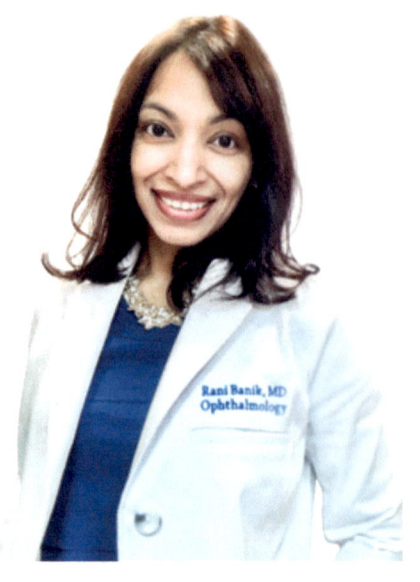

Dr. Banik's mission is to educate the public and her colleagues about eye-smart nutrition and lifestyle choices to prevent vision loss and achieve better overall health and quality of life.

Dr. Banik is often featured as an eye health expert in the media; she has been interviewed by the New York Times, Good Morning America, CBS, NBC, ABC, and many other television and radio programs. She has been an expert guest on over 75 podcasts.

"Beyond Carrots" is Dr. Banik's first book. Her second book, "Beyond Leafy Greens - The Macular Degeneration Solution" will be released soon. Be sure to connect with Dr. Banik on social media via her Facebook group, EnVision Health, or on Instagram at @dr.ranibanik for valuable tips on protecting and preserving your vision.

Made in United States
Troutdale, OR
11/28/2023